Essential Atlas

of Physiology

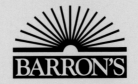

BARRON'S

First edition for the United States, its territories and
dependencies, and Canada published in 2005 by
Barron's Educational Series, Inc.

Copyright © of English-language translation 2005
by Barron's Educational Series, Inc.

Original title of the book in Spanish: *Atlas Básico de Fisiología*
Copyright © 2003 by Parramón Ediciones, S.A.—World Rights
Published by Parramón Ediciones, S.A., Barcelona, Spain

Author: Parramón's Editorial Team
Illustrations: Parramón's Editorial Team
Text: Adolfo Cassan

English translation by Marcela Estibill

All inquiries should be addressed to:
Barron's Educational Series, Inc.
250 Wireless Boulevard
Hauppauge, NY 11788
www.barronseduc.com

ISBN-13: 978-0-7641-3093-9
ISBN-10: 0-7641-3093-5

Library of Congress Catalog Card Number 2004110792

Printed in Spain
9 8 7

FOREWORD

The *Essential Atlas of Physiology* offers readers a wonderful opportunity to know the workings of the human body. It is, then, a very useful tool to access the wonders of our bodies, compared so many times to a machine, although much more complex than any device ever designed by humans.

The different chapters in this work are a complete summary of human physiology. There are many diagrams and simplified pictures, which are nonetheless accurate, depicting the main features of the different systems in our bodies. These illustrations are the core of this book, and they are complemented with different explanations and notes to facilitate the main concepts, and an index to help you find a subject easily.

When we started the edition of this atlas of physiology, we set as our goal to bring about a practical and educational work, which is useful and accessible, scientifically accurate, and also clear and entertaining. We hope our readers find that our goals have been met.

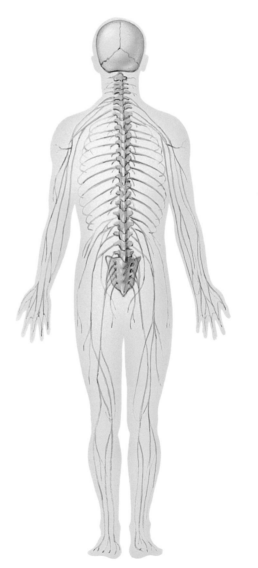

TABLE OF CONTENTS

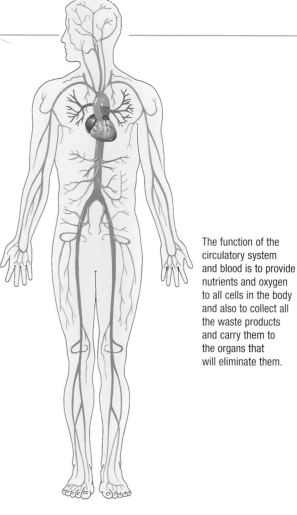

The function of the circulatory system and blood is to provide nutrients and oxygen to all cells in the body and also to collect all the waste products and carry them to the organs that will eliminate them.

PHYSIOLOGY

Physiology is the science that studies the **functioning** of living organisms, i.e., the many biological processes taking place in cells, tissues, and systems. It also studies the numerous interrelations between all the components and the control mechanisms that allow a coordinated activity. The name of this science comes from the Greek *phýsis*, meaning natural order, and *logy*, meaning study or science.

Above all, it is important to point out that physiology is closely related to other scientific disciplines, such as **anatomy**, which describes the structure of the organism and which is supported by chemistry and physics, because life is made of physiochemical processes.

And, of course, it is an important part of **medicine**, since it isn't until you understand the normal function of the body that you can comprehend its alterations and the mechanisms that produce them to be able to determine the most adequate remedy to solve disorders and to stay healthy. The branch that studies this is pathophysiology.

Some branches of physiology focus on the study of more simple living organisms, plants and animals, because, although there are multiple similarities, there are significant differences.

In this work, we will refer exclusively to **human physiology**, the oldest branch of this science. It is convenient to start by reviewing the history of this scientific discipline, because that will help us to better understand its purposes and scope.

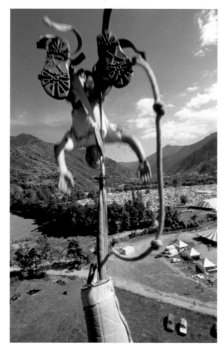

Strong emotions like those caused by "extreme" sports make the body produce certain hormones such as adrenaline.

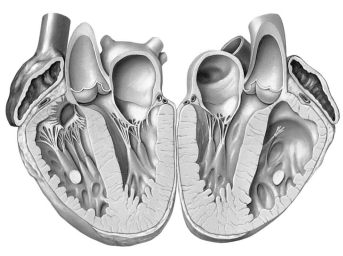

The heart is a hollow muscle that pumps blood to the whole body tirelessly. It is estimated that the heart of a 70 year old person has beaten over 2,500 million times.

FIRST STEPS IN PHYSIOLOGY

Although in the beginning physiology was considered only a part of medicine and did not develop as an independent science until the nineteenth century, it has a long history. In ancient China, they tried to explain the way the organism worked, although back then knowledge was based on **speculation** rather than research. The same happened in ancient Greece. Actually, the first data of this discipline correspond to the studies done by the Alexandrian physician **Herophylus of Chalcedon** in the year 300 B.C. He dissected many human cadavers of criminals, and, besides laying the foundations for anatomy, he tried to explain the workings of the heart and the circulatory system.

In the second century A.D. (129–201), the Greek physician **Galen** laid the foundations for what would later be experimental physiology, with his research based on dissections of animals. Among his achievements is that he demonstrated that arteries are full of blood and not air, as was thought 400 years earlier, that kidneys produce urine, and that the brain controls the vocal cords through the larynx nerves.

Although the contributions of these admirable scientists had a lot of inaccuracies, the truth is that they influenced the teaching and the practice of medicine during many centuries.

Much time had to go by and it wasn't until after the Middle Ages that knowledge in this field advanced. In the sixteenth century, some important studies were made and this was when the term "physiology" was coined; it appeared for the first time in a book published in 1548 by French physician **Jean Fernel** (1497–1558). In it the prevalent theories of medicine were presented in themes such as blood circulation, digestion, or breathing. Some were wrong theories, which eventually were refuted in the following century.

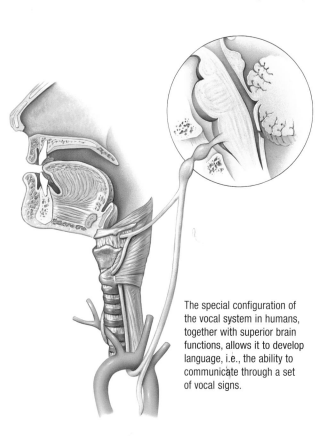

The special configuration of the vocal system in humans, together with superior brain functions, allows it to develop language, i.e., the ability to communicate through a set of vocal signs.

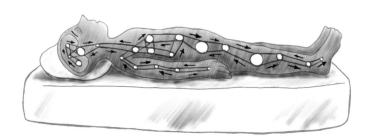

Even during sleep and rest, the different systems and organs of our body continue working in an autonomous and efficient way.

MODERN PHYSIOLOGY

"Modern physiology" was really born in the seventeenth century. It was the English physician **William Harvey** (1578–1657) who discovered and described the mechanism of blood circulation correctly. Although from our present day perspective, it may seem obvious, until then it was not known that the heart acts as a device pumping blood to all blood vessels so that it goes through the body. This discovery initially met with disbelief, but it was a milestone in the history of physiology because it questioned already accepted theories, and it encouraged research on the functioning of the body.

Great progress was achieved in the field of physics and chemistry throughout the eighteenth century and that allowed great advances in physiology. It was about this time when important phenomena were described, such as the gas exchange that takes place in the lungs between air and blood, gastric juice activity during digestion, or the electrical mechanism of muscle contractions. Undoubtedly these contributions to physiology meant an enormous advance in knowledge, although it was only partial.

CONTEMPORARY KNOWLEDGE

An important figure appears in the nineteenth century: physiologist **Claude Bernard** (1813–1878), creator of an experimental method to acquire knowledge based on the formulation of a hypothesis, observation, and the formulation of doubts, proofs, and confirmations. Bernard studied the metabolism of carbon hydrates, digestion in human beings, the activity of the autonomous nervous system and

many other matters. Through his publications, he became the spokesman of physiological knowledge of his time. His greatest contribution was to establish the principle that living organisms are never at rest but instead are going through continuous changes with the objective of maintaining internal balance. The basis for health, as proposed by Bernard, is when the body manages to keep this balance. The principles stated by this great scientist were confirmed over time, and they were also expended. During the twentieth century, discoveries have been occurring one after the other, especially because of technological progress, developments in biochemistry, and advances in genetics. These factors have provided an enormous boost for physiology and allow us to have, in the beginning of the twenty-first century, a thorough knowledge of the human body.

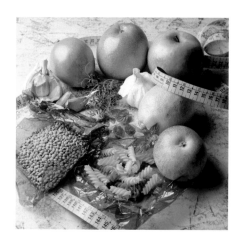

To have our bodies working properly, it is essential to have good eating habits.

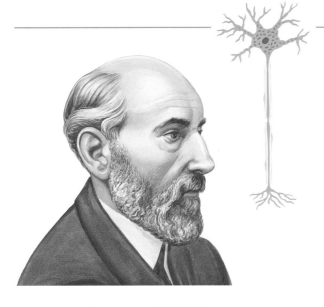

Many physicians and scientists have studied the human body. Santiago Ramón y Cajal (1852–1934) from Spain, for example, carried out important research on human nervous tissue, and especially on neurons.

THE PARTS OF A WHOLE

Human physiology covers, as it has been said, a broad field. Nowadays we can know accurately, among other things, the mechanisms by which the constant exchange of matter and energy is produced between the body and the outside world, an important factor in life. We also know the necessary mechanisms for getting those resources, such as digestion, that allow us to assimilate basic nutrients in food, or breathing to obtain oxygen. Cells use oxygen as fuel for metabolic reactions that provide them with energy.

And, much more, because physiology tries to explain in great detail the function of each and every one of the parts of our bodies. It tries to explain the heart, which acts as a pump pushing blood to an intricate network of blood vessels so that blood goes through the whole body, carrying nutrients and oxygen to tissues; kidneys, which filter blood tirelessly to eliminate, through urine, metabolic waste; the musculoskeletal system, which allows us to move in everyday life; the endocrine system, which, through hormones, regulates the function of the whole body; the nervous system, which controls all organic reactions and is also responsible for higher mental functions.

However, it is worth mentioning that although the human body is made up of different systems, it works as a unit. To be alive and healthy, it is extremely important that all tissues and organs keep a perfectly coordinated activity, because they are, in great part, interdependent in their functions.

Given what has been said, and this must be clearly understood, the division of the body in systems is, in a certain way, artificial and for teaching purposes, because it helps to understand, partially, the work of each part of the body. For this reason, even though this book constantly refers to the interrelations between the different areas, it will review each and every system of the human body separately.

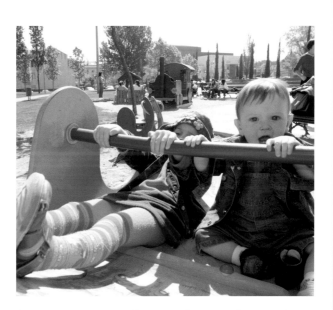

The human being, in spite of being the only intelligent living organism, is one of the animals who takes longer to complete the learning process.

A PERFECT MACHINE

The different systems in our bodies have specific missions and perform coordinated activity. They are like the parts in a machine but with an important difference: they can regenerate themselves, and they can repair the damage when there is a malfunction.

Nervous System

It is like a huge computer, it automatically controls the functioning of the whole body, it allows us to perform voluntary actions. Specifically, the brain is the center of our intellectual and emotional activities

Circulatory System

It is like a transportation system, it carries blood throughout the body to provide the tissues with the necessary nutrients and oxygen, and it takes the metabolic waste to the purifying organs

Digestive System

It processes food to provide the body with the elements to obtain the materials and the energy needed by the different tissues to generate their components and perform their functions

Blood

It travels throughout the body carrying the substances needed by cells in all tissues to perform their activity, and it carries the waste products to the purifying organs

Reproductive System

It allows us to develop a sexual life, and it is responsible for the wonderful process of procreation of new beings

Musculoskeletal System

Bones make up the shell of the body, and because of the action of muscles and joints, our bodies can move

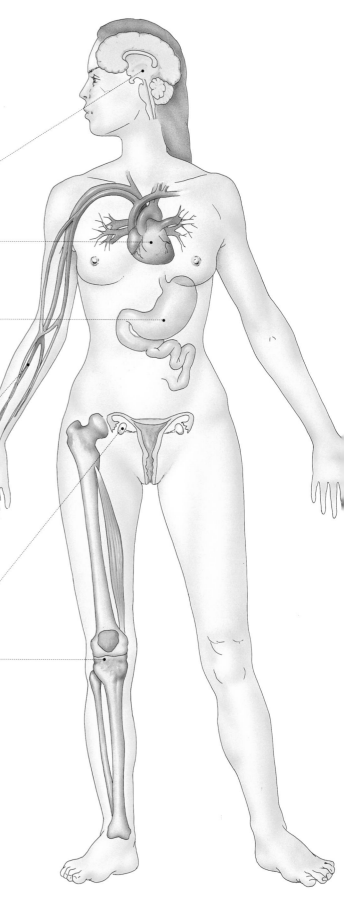

CONSTANT RENOVATION

Unlike machines, the elements that are part of the human being are renewed constantly: every minute billions of cells are formed in our bodies to replace those that have been damaged.

Introduction

A Perfect Machine

Skin

Digestive System

Nutrition

Respiratory System

Circulatory System and Blood

Nervous System

Musculoskeletal System

Urinary System

Endocrine System

Immune System

The Senses

Genetics

Reproductive System

Human Development

Index

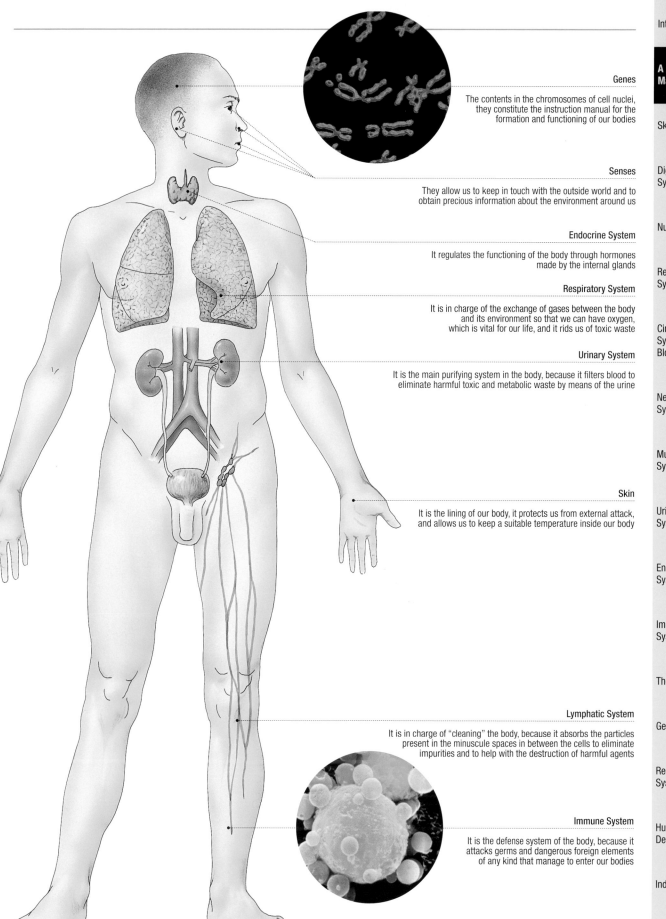

Genes

The contents in the chromosomes of cell nuclei, they constitute the instruction manual for the formation and functioning of our bodies

Senses

They allow us to keep in touch with the outside world and to obtain precious information about the environment around us

Endocrine System

It regulates the functioning of the body through hormones made by the internal glands

Respiratory System

It is in charge of the exchange of gases between the body and its environment so that we can have oxygen, which is vital for our life, and it rids us of toxic waste

Urinary System

It is the main purifying system in the body, because it filters blood to eliminate harmful toxic and metabolic waste by means of the urine

Skin

It is the lining of our body, it protects us from external attack, and allows us to keep a suitable temperature inside our body

Lymphatic System

It is in charge of "cleaning" the body, because it absorbs the particles present in the minuscule spaces in between the cells to eliminate impurities and to help with the destruction of harmful agents

Immune System

It is the defense system of the body, because it attacks germs and dangerous foreign elements of any kind that manage to enter our bodies

THE SKIN, OUR FIRST GARMENT

The skin is a thick **membrane**, resistant and flexible, with many connected structures (sweat glands, sensitive receptors, hair follicles, and nails) and it constitutes the **body's protective layer**, although it performs other important functions.

FUNCTIONS OF THE SKIN

Three distinct layers form the skin, one on top of the other (epidermis, dermis, and hypodermis). The main function of the skin is to act as a **protective barrier**, blocking the passage into the body of germs, harmful chemicals, or harmful agents present in the environment. It also helps in the regulation of body temperature, and, internally, it cushions the effects of mechanical stresses, it constitutes an important reservoir of energy, and it acts as a **sensory organ**.

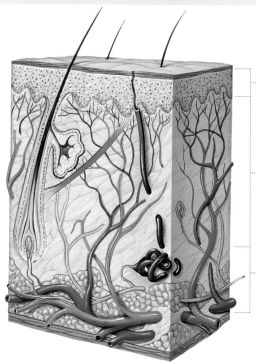

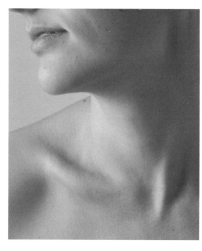

Acne (from the Greek *acme*, point) has a palliative treatment.

In an adult, the skin has a total area of 1.5 to 2 m², and just the dermis and epidermis weigh approximately 4 kg.

STRUCTURE OF THE SKIN

Epidermis

It is the superficial layer formed by various layers of epithelium cells in direct contact with the outside world

Dermis

It is the intermediate layer formed by cells and fibers of connective tissue, where the various skin appendages are found, with plenty of vascularization and a rich sensitive innervation

Hypodermis

It is the deepest layer, with different thicknesses in different parts of the body. It is basically made of fat tissue, with many fat cells, which constitute the main reservoir of energy in the body and act as insulation

REGENERATION OF THE EPIDERMIS

The epidermis experiences a constant renovation process. Surface cells are exposed to the wear and tear that comes with environmental contact and the multiple stresses that implies. They continually flake off and are replaced by other cells from deep beneath. Actually, base cells multiply endlessly and the new cells push the ones on top toward the surface. They go through various layers, suffering changes and losing vitality, until they reach the horny layer. After a while, these cells come off. This process takes between 20 and 30 days; it can be stated that we change epidermis each month.

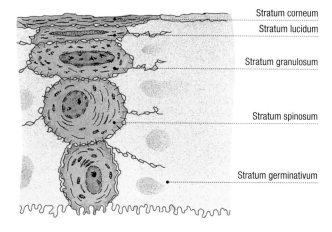

SOME SKIN DISORDERS

Albinism: A pigmentation disorder characterized by scarcity or absence of coloration in skin, hair, or eyes

Acne: A common disorder in adolescence, characterized by pimples or blackheads

Dermatitis: Skin inflammation

Psoriasis: A chronic disorder characterized by the formation of red plates covered by white flakes that come off

Warts: Small tumors in the epidermis caused by a viral infection

THE LAYERS OF THE EPIDERMIS

Stratum corneum
Stratum lucidum
Stratum granulosum
Stratum spinosum
Stratum germinativum

SCARRING

Introduction

A Perfect Machine

Skin

Digestive System

Nutrition

Respiratory System

Circulatory System and Blood

Nervous System

Musculoskeletal System

Urinary System

Endocrine System

Immune System

The Senses

Genetics

Reproductive System

Human Development

Index

THE SCARRING PROCESS

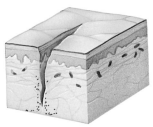

the borders of the wound are separated

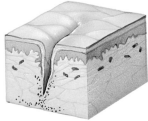

from the borders, a fibrous tissue spreads, filling the void

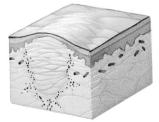

the continuation of the epidermis is reestablished at the bottom of the wound

the fibrous tissue pushes the epidermis toward the surface

The **consequences of a wound** in the skin depend on the depth of the injury. If only the epidermis is affected, as happens with a scrape, tissue regenerates, starting from the basal layer, and no visible marks are left. However, when the dermis is also affected, as happens with a cut, there is a gap and both borders of the wound separate and the **scarring process** starts. From the borders **granulation tissue**, made up of cells and connective fibers, little by little fills the empty spaces and restores the continuity of the epidermis, and finally covers the wound. However, because the epidermis layer of the area is thinner than normal and the connective tissue that repairs the wound does not have the same structure as the original dermis, a pink mark is left, at first, which then turns white, and this is what we call a scar.

SKIN COLORATION

The color of the skin depends on a pigment called **melanin**, whose function is to absorb solar radiations and to prevent them from entering the body where they would be harmful. Some specialized cells, **melanocytes**, present deep in the epidermis produce pigment. Their number and degree of activity are regulated by **hormonal** and **genetic** factors. This would explain the diverse skin coloration of individuals from different races and of each person, in particular. The main stimulus for the production of melanin corresponds to sun exposure, which results in the sun-tanning phenomenon.

MELANOCYTE

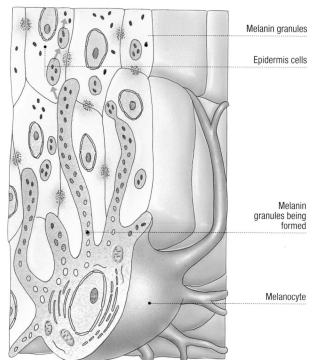

Melanin granules

Epidermis cells

Melanin granules being formed

Melanocyte

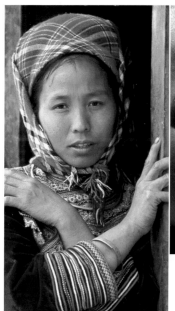

Skin pigmentation protects us from solar radiations, although the darker the skin, the better the protection.

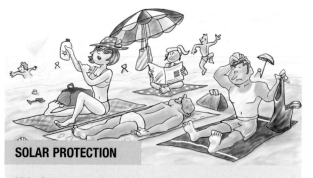

SOLAR PROTECTION

Melanin protects us from solar radiations, and its production increases when we sunbathe. For this reason, we tan during summer. But prolonged solar exposure should be avoided. We may suffer sunburn if we do not sunbathe gradually and properly protected.

REGULATION OF BODY TEMPERATURE

THERMOREGULATION

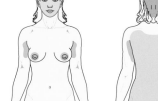

The skin plays an important role in **thermoregulation**, i.e., keeping the body at a constant temperature of 98.6°F. When it is cold, the subcutaneous blood vessels contract, to prevent the blood circulating near the surface of the body from getting cold. When the temperature outside is high, the vessels dilate to facilitate heat loss, which is also aided by the evaporation of sweat.

Contraction of piloerector muscle

Decrease in sweating

Contraction of skin capillaries

Dilatation of skin pores

Increase in sweating

Dilatation of skin capillaries

Sweat is odorless until bacteria present on the surface of the body start acting on its components; regular hygiene prevents unpleasant odors.

DISTRIBUTION OF SWEAT GLANDS IN THE BODY

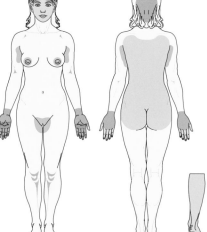

Eccrine Glands:

- Over 300/cm²
- Over 200/cm²
- Over 100/cm²
- Less than 100/cm²
- **Apocrine glands**

SWEAT GLANDS

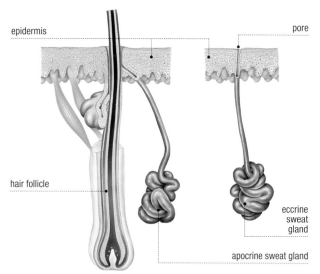

epidermis

pore

hair follicle

eccrine sweat gland

apocrine sweat gland

SWEAT

Sweat is the **secretion** of sweat glands and is basically made up of water that has small amounts of dissolved salts and various chemicals coming from metabolism. There are two types of sweat glands: **eccrine** and **apocrine** glands. Eccrine glands are most numerous and open into the pores on the surface of the skin. Apocrine glands direct their secretions to a hair follicle. Sweat gland activity, controlled by the autonomous nervous system, contributes to regulate body temperature because the evaporation of sweat has a refreshing effect on the skin.

PSYCHOLOGICAL STIMULI

Many mental stimuli, such as **nervousness** and **fear**, can cause a large amount of sweat, although it is only evident on the palms of our hands and on the soles of our feet. These secretions do not have any apparent function and are related to primitive reflex mechanisms that allow the body to adapt to extreme conditions.

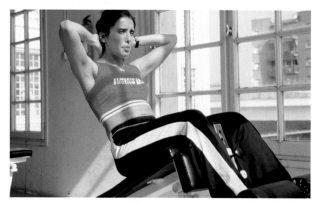

A minimum of half a liter of sweat is produced each day, which is barely noticeable, but that amount can markedly increase in a hot environment and when you exercise.

SEBACEOUS GLANDS

The sebaceous glands are distributed along the surface of the body but are more numerous on the face, chest, back, and genital area. They produce a fatty secretion that forms a protective layer on the epidermis and lubricates the hairs. Sebum has a **protective function**, because it gets mixed with the scaling from the epidermis and with sweat. It constitutes an acidic fatty layer that, among other things, slows down the growth of germs on the skin surface. When room temperature is low, the sebaceous secretion becomes harder and makes evaporation of sweat more difficult, and by doing so helps to maintain body temperature.

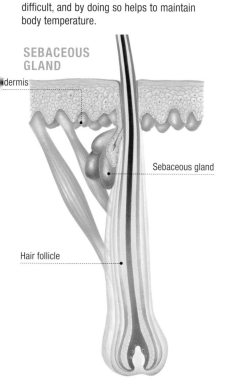

SEBACEOUS GLAND

Epidermis

Sebaceous gland

Hair follicle

HAIR GROWTH

Each hair on the body grows from a hair follicle, more specifically, from the deepest part of it, called the **germinative matrix**, where cells fill up with a fibrous protein called **keratin** and then die, constituting the hair shaft that comes out and ends up outside the skin. Throughout life, hairs go through the **anagen stage**, which lasts approximately 3 years, the **telogen stage** during which the follicle activity stops for a few weeks, **and the catagen stage**, which lasts a few months and after which a new hair starts growing, pushing the old hair until the latter falls out.

Hair grows at different speeds, between 0.1–0.5 mm a day, depending on the individual.

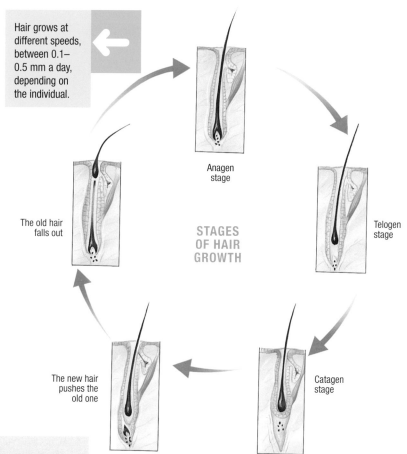

Anagen stage

Telogen stage

Catagen stage

The new hair pushes the old one

The old hair falls out

STAGES OF HAIR GROWTH

NAIL GROWTH

Nails are **thin** but **hard** and resistant **sheets** whose function is to **protect** the last phalange of fingers and toes. They are also useful in performing actions that require some precision, as pincer-like grabbing, folding, or separating. Their structure is similar to that of hair, because they are mostly made up of keratin and are produced by the epidermis. Growth occurs in the root, which is hidden from view. There, the cells of the stratum corneum produce a very hard keratin that slides on the nail bed forming a sheet, which is the nail. Although the speed of nail growth varies depending on the individual, it is estimated at about 0.1 mm in one day.

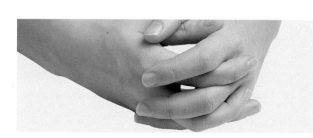

NAIL STRUCTURE

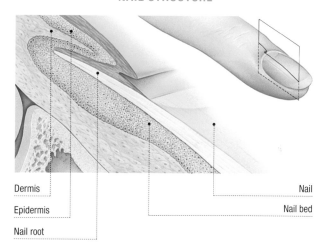

Dermis

Epidermis

Nail root

Nail

Nail bed

THE DIGESTIVE SYSTEM

The digestive system is in charge of **transforming food** by making it undergo a series of mechanical and chemical processes to free its basic components, which are then absorbed into the blood and transported throughout the body in order for the body to obtain materials and energy destined to form tissue and guarantee the vital functions.

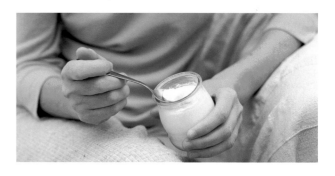

THE DIGESTIVE TUBE

Diagrammatically, the digestive system is formed by a **long tube**, which goes through the body from the mouth to the anus. Each section constitutes an **organ**, with its own function, but all the actions of the tube are perfectly coordinated to **digest the food** that follows the path, absorb basic nutrients resulting from the digestive process, and finally get rid of the residues that are not assimilated.

Mouth

In charge of crushing the food and submitting it to the action of saliva, preparing the resulting bolus for its passage through the digestive tube

Pharynx

Takes part in swallowing

Esophagus

Carries the bolus from the throat to the stomach

Liver

Produces bile, needed for digesting fats and has different roles in metabolism, such as rendering toxic products inactive

Gallbladder

Stores the bile produced in the liver and after meals; pours it in the duodenum

Duodenum

The first section of the small intestine, where food is digested by action of the intestinal enzymes, pancreatic juice, and bile to obtain the basic nutrients

Large intestine

Digestion and assimilation of nutrients ends in the colon, where the water from the bolus gets absorbed and the residues are turned into fecal matter

Small intestine

In its passage through the small intestine, nutrients are absorbed into the blood to get distributed to the whole body

Rectum

The last portion of the large intestine stores the residues of the digestive process to be pushed out through defecation

Stomach

Stores the bolus and puts it under the powerful corrosive action of gastric juices and then sends it, once it becomes a semiliquid substance, into the small intestine

Pancreas

Produces the pancreatic juice made of digestive enzymes essential for digesting food

DIGESTION TIME

How long is it from the time we eat food until we evacuate it? As a matter of fact, the time between one and the other varies, because it depends on numerous factors, among them, the composition of food. However, on average, the approximate time food stays in each portion of the digestive tube is the following:

- **Mouth:** 1–2 minutes
- **Esophagus:** seconds
- **Stomach:** 2–4 hours
- **Small intestine:** 2–4 hours
- **Large intestine:** 10–48 hours

HUNGER AND SATISFACTION

The feeling of appetite is regulated by two nervous centers located in the hypothalamus, the **center of hunger** and the **center of satisfaction**, whose stimulation depends on the information from the stomach and the senses. When the stomach stays empty for a long time, the hunger center activates and the **desire to eat** emerges, just as happens when we see or smell some delicious food. When the stomach is full, the center of satisfaction receives the stimulus, so the desire to eat vanishes.

HUNGER AND SATISFACTION CENTERS

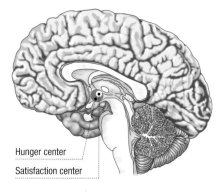

Hunger center

Satisfaction center

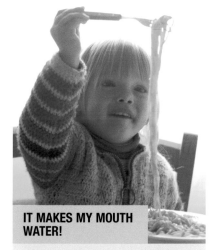

IT MAKES MY MOUTH WATER!

Why is it that we produce saliva sometimes without tasting food, when we see a delicious dish, when we smell it, or even when we think about it? Because those stimuli are interpreted by the nervous nuclei of the encephalon that controls saliva production as if we were going to eat the food we are seeing, smelling, or imagining. It can be said that when faced with an attractive or a delicious dish, the digestion process begins before we start eating.

MASTICATION

Chewing is a **reflex action** in which powerful chewing muscles move the jaw up and down, teeth cut and crush food, saliva moistens the food fragments and the tongue. Finally, with the help of lips and cheeks, it turns a solid product into a semiliquid mixture, the **bolus**. Actually, it starts as a voluntary action, since the brain sends the order to the chewing muscles to contract, but it then turns into an automatic action. When the food enters into contact with the palate and the surface of the mouth, a muscle relaxation occurs and the lower jaw falls. This is followed by a bouncing effect and the muscles contract, firmly pulling up the jaw to make it tighten against the upper jaw. This cycle repeats without our thinking about it until food has been swallowed entirely.

STRUCTURES INVOLVED IN CHEWING

Upper jaw

Buccinator muscle

Teeth

Tongue

Parotid gland

Masseter muscle

Sublingual gland

Submandibular gland

Lower jaw or mandible

SALIVARY GLANDS

Along the oral cavity, there are many small glands that produce small amounts of saliva almost constantly. The main three pairs that drain their secretions inside the mouth are the **parotid glands**, the **submandibular glands**, and the **sublingual glands**. These are the glands that, controlled by the autonomous nervous system, produce bigger amounts of saliva when we eat.

SALIVARY FUNCTION

Saliva moistens food to ease chewing, but that is not its only objective. It also has an antiseptic effect, because it contains white cells and enzymes that act against many bacteria that can penetrate the mouth. It also has a digestive enzyme, which starts digesting starches in the mouth. It is important in speech, because keeping the lips and mouth moistened helps the articulation of words.

MY MOUTH IS DRY!

The production of saliva is controlled by the **autonomous nervous system** that regulates in an automatic way various organic functions. But the autonomous nervous system is divided into two areas with opposing actions, called the **parasympathetic** and **sympathetic**. The former dominates when we are at rest, the latter activates in alert situations, when we are nervous or feel fear. The activation of the sympathetic system, among other things, interrupts the secretion of saliva. That is why we notice our mouths dry when we face a situation that makes us anxious.

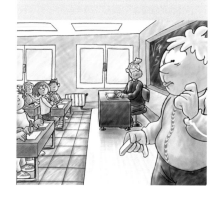

TEETH

Teeth are **hard** and **resistant pieces** that are inserted in the upper and lower jaws. Their job is to **cut**, **tear**, and **crush food**. There are three easily identifiable parts in each tooth: the **crown**, the visible part that sticks out from the gum, the **dental neck**, the part in the middle covered by the gum, and the **root**, the internal part inserted in the jaw bone. The crown is formed on the outside by **enamel**, the hardest tissue in the body. Underneath is a hard layer of **dentine**, a less hard tissue that also forms the root. In the center of the tooth there is a cavity, the **pulp**, which is full of a softer tissue that contains blood vessels and nerves that enter through the root of the tooth.

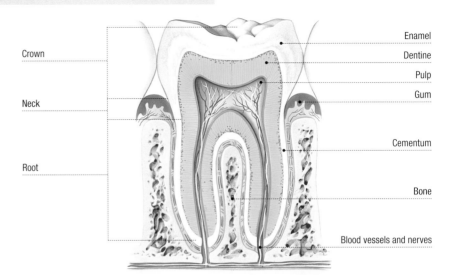

Crown
Neck
Root

Enamel
Dentine
Pulp
Gum
Cementum
Bone
Blood vessels and nerves

FUNCTIONS OF TEETH

Humans have four types of teeth, each one with a particular shape and a specific function.

The **incisors** are foremost and have the shape of a shovel or chisel with a sharp edge and have only one root. They act like metal shears and their task is to cut and break food.

The **canine** teeth are located behind the incisors and are a little bigger. They have a pointy crown and one longer root. Their job is to tear elastic or hard food.

The **premolars** are behind the canines. They have a more voluminous crown with two protuberances and a central depression. They have one root. They are in charge of crushing food.

The **molars** are rearmost, located on both ends of the set of teeth. They have a square crown with a flat surface that has four prominences or apexes and their roots divide into two or three branches. They also crush or grind hard food.

TEETHING

Humans have two sets of teeth throughout life: **deciduous** teeth, made up of 20 **baby teeth**, which after a few years fall out to allow room for a set of **permanent teeth** made up of 32 teeth, which will never be replaced. The **primary teething**, formed by eight incisors, four canines, and eight molars starts at about six months of age and finishes at about $2\frac{1}{2}$ years of age or a little later. These teeth fall out on their own, starting from age six, and leave their place for the permanent teeth. The **secondary teething**, formed by eight premolars and twelve molars, starts at about age six or seven and ends between ages sixteen and thirty.

TYPES OF TEETH

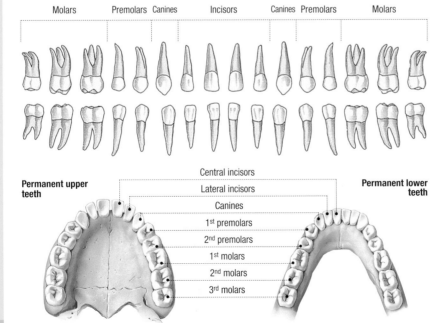

Molars   Premolars Canines   Incisors   Canines Premolars   Molars

Permanent upper teeth

Central incisors
Lateral incisors
Canines
1st premolars
2nd premolars
1st molars
2nd molars
3rd molars

Permanent lower teeth

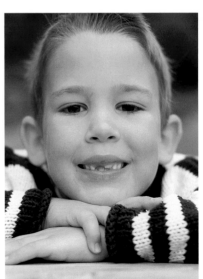

Baby teeth fall out at age six or seven.

ERUPTION OF BABY TEETH (Figures in months)

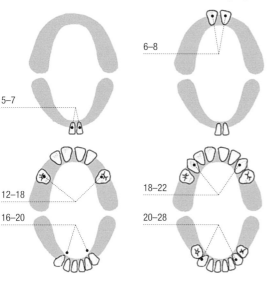

6–8

8–11

7–10

5–7

12–18

18–22

22–30

16–20

20–28

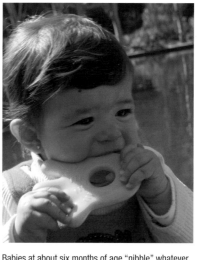

Babies at about six months of age "nibble" whatever they can reach to relieve the pain that is produced by the first set of teeth breaking out.

WISDOM TEETH

The third molars are also known as **wisdom teeth**, a popular name that relates to the fact that they appear between ages 16 and 25 years, when a person supposedly is wise. However, many people never get these teeth because they do not have enough room for them. This fact seems to be related to the evolution of humans: nowadays jawbones tend to develop less, maybe as a consequence of the changes in the items we eat, which do not require such intense chewing as the food primitive humans ate. As a matter of fact, the absence of wisdom teeth does not affect chewing much, because the location of these teeth, at the ends of the set of teeth, makes them less efficient.

ERUPTION OF PERMANENT TEETH
(Figures in years)

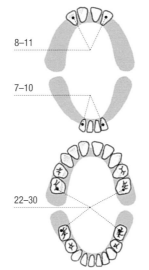

7–8

8–9

11–12

10–11

10–12

6–7

12–13

16–25

16–25

12–13

6–7

11–13

10–12

9–11

7–8

6–7

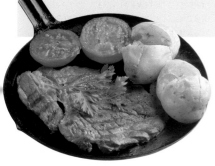

Without wisdom teeth, you can still perfectly crush food like meat.

Canines are also called **canine teeth** and molars are also known as **molar teeth**.

BABY TEETH	COME OUT		FALL OUT	
	Lower	Upper	Lower	Upper
Central incisors	5–7 months	6–8 months	6–7 years old	7–8 years old
Lateral incisors	8–10 months	8–12 months	7–8 years old	8–9 years old
Canine teeth	14–18 months	16–20 months	9–11 years old	11–12 years old
1st Molars	12–18 months	12–18 months	10–11 years old	10–12 years old
2nd Molars	20–28 months	22–30 months	10–12 years old	11–13 years old
PERMANENT TEETH				
Central incisors	6–8 years old	7–9 years old		
Lateral incisors	7–8 years old	8–10 years old		
Canine teeth	9–11 years old	11–13 years old		
1st Premolars	10–12 years old	10–12 years old		
2nd Premolars	11–13 years old	10–12 years old		
1st Molars	6–7 years old	6–7 years old		
2nd Molars	11–13 years old	11–13 years old		
3rd Molars	16–25 years old	16–25 years old		

DEGLUTITION

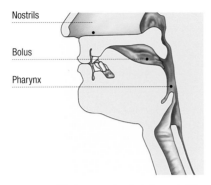

The tongue pushes the bolus against the palate and toward the pharynx

Nostrils
Bolus
Pharynx

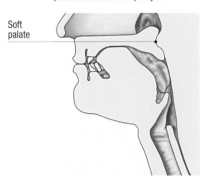

The soft palate goes up to keep the bolus from going into the nostrils

Soft palate

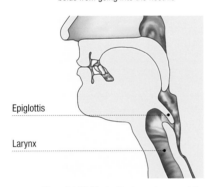

The epiglottis blocks the larynx to prevent the bolus from going to the breathing passages

Epiglottis
Larynx

The **act of swallowing** is a complex mechanism by which the bolus goes from the mouth, through the pharynx and the esophagus, to the stomach. This action, which starts voluntarily and then turns into an automatic action, requires a correct coordination of the movements of various parts of the body, because different obstacles must be overcome. When the bolus goes through the pharynx, it is necessary that the **soft palate** go up to prevent it from going into the nostrils. In the same way, the **epiglottis** inclines to prevent the bolus from going into the breathing passages. Next, the **upper esophageal sphincter**, a muscular valve that keeps the entrance to the esophagus closed, has to open so that air does not go into the digestive tube. Then the **lower esophageal sphincter**, which under normal conditions keeps the opening to the stomach closed to prevent the passing of gastric juice toward the mouth, must open. Fortunately, we do not have to think of all these actions, because they happen as a **reflex** from the moment the food enters the pharynx.

DEGLUTITION MECHANISM

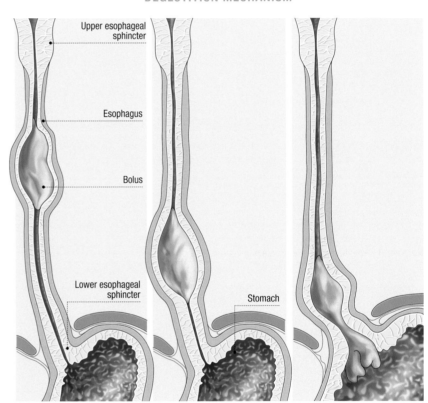

Upper esophageal sphincter
Esophagus
Bolus
Lower esophageal sphincter
Stomach

Upper esophageal sphincter opens to allow the bolus to enter the esophagus.

The muscles of the walls of the esophagus contract in sequence to push the bolus toward the stomach.

Lower esophageal sphincter opens to allow the bolus to enter the stomach.

The passing of the bolus from the mouth to the stomach happens because of the various muscles of the pharynx and the esophagus, not simply gravity; that is why it is possible to swallow if we are lying down.

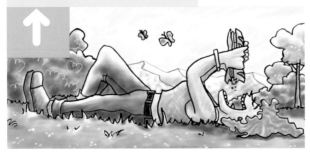

ROLE OF THE STOMACH

The stomach's role is to **store** the eaten food temporarily so that, little by little, it reaches the small intestine and continues its passage through the digestive tube in good condition to be better used. While in the stomach, the bolus is **mixed** and **crushed** due to the powerful contractions of the muscle walls. It is also subjected to the action of the gastric juices, produced by the mucosa that covers the inner surface of the stomach, turning into a liquefied mass called **chyme**, which will later be further affected by the action of the digestive agents. The **pylorus** is a **muscular valve** that regulates the passage of the gastric content into the small intestine.

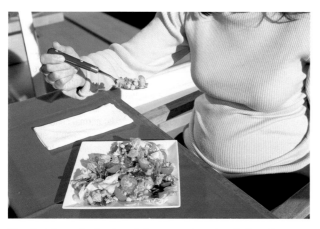

When the bolus reaches the stomach, the movements produced in the walls move the contents. These gastric movements intensify to crush the food while the pylorus, the valve that connects the stomach with the small intestine, stays closed. When the food has turned into a semifluid mass, the valve opens, allowing a small amount of the contents into the small intestine. Finally, the valve closes and the process repeats until the stomach empties.

GASTRIC SECRETION

The inner wall of the stomach is covered by a mucous layer that has numerous tiny glands in charge of secreting substances that make up the **gastric juice**. One of its main components is **pepsin**, an enzyme whose job consists of digesting proteins, i.e., breaking up the nutrients and releasing a basic unit—the amino acid—so that later it can be absorbed by the intestine. Another fundamental component is **hydrochloric acid (HCl)**, which is needed to activate pepsin. Hydrochloric acid is also a **powerful corrosive** that softens food and is capable of destroying germs. Some glands in the gastric walls also secrete mucus and bicarbonate, forming a thin layer on the internal surface of the stomach to protect the organ against the corrosive action of hydrochloric acid.

SECRETION OF GASTRIC JUICE

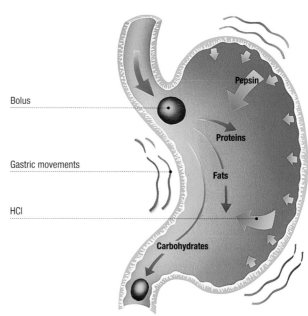

Bolus

Gastric movements

HCl

Pepsin

Proteins

Fats

Carbohydrates

REGULATION OF GASTRIC SECRETION

Gastric juice is being produced continuously, but it intensifies when you eat. As a matter of fact, gastric secretion increases simply by thinking of eating and after seeing, smelling, or tasting food, because the nervous system is always ready for the imminent arrival of food in the stomach, and it tells the stomach glands to get active. It also stimulates gastric secretion of a hormone called **gastrin**. This hormone is released when the stomach gets distended, as it gets full of food, and also when amino acids are released due to the fractionation of proteins in the small intestine. So, the secretion of gastric juice increases even before tasting food, and it intensifies when the stomach is full, especially when the food has a bigger proportion of proteins.

FACTORS REGULATING GASTRIC SECRETION

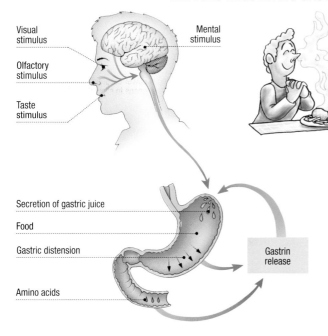

Visual stimulus

Olfactory stimulus

Taste stimulus

Mental stimulus

Secretion of gastric juice

Food

Gastric distension

Amino acids

Gastrin release

MAIN STOMACH DISEASES

Gastritis: Inflammation of the stomach inner mucosa, which causes digestive changes and abdominal discomfort.

Gastric ulcer: Erosion of the mucosa that covers the inside of the stomach. It is manifested by heartburn and abdominal pain; it usually scars in a few weeks, but it tends to reappear periodically.

Stomach cancer: Malignant tumor that grows in the stomach wall.

CHARACTERISTICS OF THE SMALL INTESTINE

CROSS SECTION OF THE SMALL INTESTINE

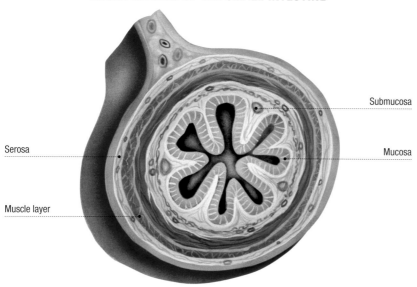

Submucosa

Serosa

Mucosa

Muscle layer

The small intestine is a tube about 7 or 8 meters long and about 3 centimeters in diameter. On its wall you can identify four layers: a **mucosa layer**, which covers the inner surface and has many glands and secreting cells; a **submucosa** located under the mucosa, which contains an extensive network of blood and lymph capillaries; a thick **muscular layer**, responsible for the motility of the organ; and a **serosa layer** that covers the tube on the outside.

ROLE OF THE SMALL INTESTINE

The **digestion** of food coming from the stomach is completed in the small intestine. There, it is broken down to its basic components, and most of the nutrients released are **absorbed** or **assimilated**. Inside the small intestine, food undergoes the **chemical action** of various enzymes. Some of these enzymes are produced by tiny glands located on the intestinal wall, and others come from the pancreas and liver. These secretions pour into the duodenum, the first section of the organ.

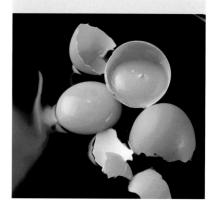

THE INTESTINAL MUCOSA

Microvilli

Blood and lymph capillaries

Intestinal villus

Villi

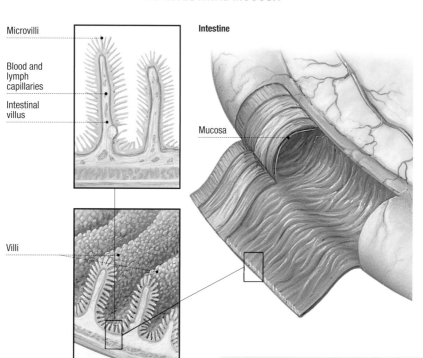

Intestine

Mucosa

If the mucosa that covers the intestine wall were to be laid out on a flat surface, it would cover an area equivalent to a soccer field.

CHARACTERISTICS OF THE INTESTINAL MUCOSA

The mucous layer covering the inside of the small intestine has some very special characteristics whose purpose is to increase the contact surface with food and thus facilitate the absorption of nutrients. On the one hand, the mucosa has small projections into the lumen of the organ, **intestinal villi**, made up of a thin layer of cells. Each one of these villi, resembling a gloved finger, has inside, small blood and lymph capillaries. The surface of the cells that form such villi have an edge similar to a brush, with numerous hair-like formations called intestinal **microvilli**, which further increase the absorption surface for nutrients.

INTESTINAL ABSORPTION

Once food has been digested by the action of the enzymes located in the lumen of the intestine, the pieces of food are so small that they can be absorbed or **assimilated**, i.e., they enter the blood and lymph vessels located inside the intestinal villi. Some molecules passively enter the gastric mucosa cells of the surface through small pores. Other molecules enter the cells through a process called **pinocytosis** (they are engulfed by the membrane and introduced in the cell). After entering the cells, the molecules come out the opposite end and reach the center of the villi, entering blood or lymph circulation.

INTESTINAL MOTILITY

The wall of the small intestine has different types of **contractions**, which facilitate the mixture of food and digestive secretions, and allow the contents to move to the large intestine. The arrival of food from the stomach causes some automatic contractions in those intestinal segments whose purpose is the **crushing** of the contents (1). There are also opposite contractions in those adjacent segments to manage a rocking movement to **mix** the contents with digestive secretions (2). And, finally, there are sequential contractions that facilitate the **passage** of contents to the large intestine (3). The opening of the **ileocecal valve** allows the passage of already digested food from the small intestine into the large intestine.

MECHANISM OF INTESTINAL ABSORPTION

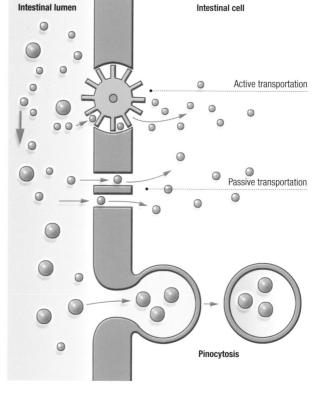

Intestinal lumen

Intestinal cell

Active transportation

Passive transportation

Pinocytosis

DIAGRAM OF INTESTINAL MOVEMENTS

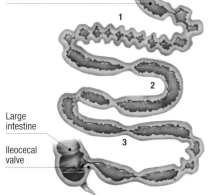

Small intestine

1

2

3

Large intestine

Ileocecal valve

The intestinal movements that cause the passage of materials along the tube are known as **peristalsis**.

FUNCTION OF THE LARGE INTESTINE

Residues are stored in the large intestine, and water is absorbed. Some salts containing very useful elements for our bodies and whose loss would be harmful are also absorbed here. As the semifluid mass from the small intestine goes through the colon, it turns into a more compact mass called a **fecal bolus**. Actually, many dead bacteria from the intestinal flora, cells flaked off the intestinal wall, and some other **organic waste** are added to this partially dried waste, all of which constitute fecal matter. The fecal bolus is stored in the rectum until this gets full, then the waste is expelled outside the body.

Fruits and vegetables, which contain a high percentage of water, are some of the foods more easily absorbed.

A milligram of fecal matter contains the residues of more than 1,500,000 bacteria from the intestinal flora.

FORMATION OF FECAL MATTER

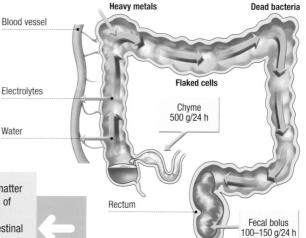

Blood vessel

Electrolytes

Water

Heavy metals

Dead bacteria

Flaked cells

Chyme
500 g/24 h

Rectum

Anus

Fecal bolus
100–150 g/24 h

Introduction

A Perfect Machine

Skin

Digestive System

Nutrition

Respiratory System

Circulatory System and Blood

Nervous System

Musculoskeletal System

Urinary System

Endocrine System

Immune System

The Senses

Genetics

Reproductive System

Human Development

Index

THE LIVER

The liver is considered an **accessory organ in the digestive system**, although it performs many important functions, which makes it one of the vital organs. The liver tissue actually has one of the most complex structures in the body. Liver cells, **hepatocytes**, are arranged in layers that form partitions around the small channels that travel the whole organ. Through these channels there are ramifications of the **hepatic artery** and the **portal vein**, vessels that carry blood to the organ and from which the liver receives the substances it must treat. There are also some small bile ducts or ductules where the hepatocytes pour the **bile** they produce.

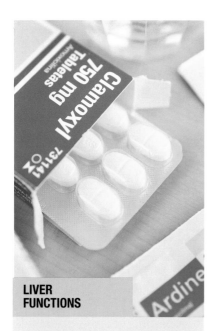

LIVER FUNCTIONS

• Producing bile, the basic element for digesting fats.

• Metabolizing nutrients absorbed in the digestive tube, an essential step for food utilization.

• Storing carbohydrates as glycogen, some minerals, and various vitamins.

• Cleansing several elements transported by blood, such as waste products (bilirubin, ammonia, etc.), hormones, and medication buildup in the body, which are toxic.

• Syntheses of several substances, especially proteins and vitamins.

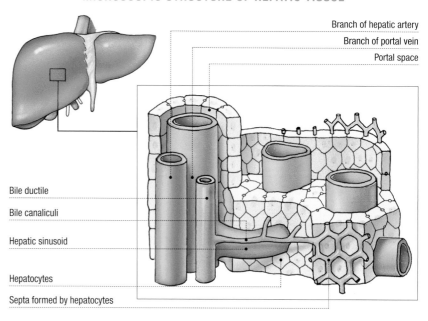

Branch of hepatic artery
Branch of portal vein
Portal space

Bile ductile
Bile canaliculi
Hepatic sinusoid
Hepatocytes
Septa formed by hepatocytes

LIVER ACTIVITY

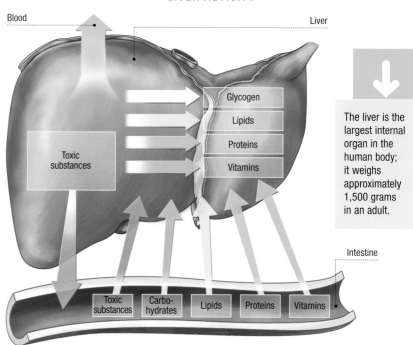

Blood

Liver

Glycogen
Lipids
Proteins
Vitamins

Toxic substances

Toxic substances | Carbo-hydrates | Lipids | Proteins | Vitamins

The liver is the largest internal organ in the human body; it weighs approximately 1,500 grams in an adult.

Intestine

BILE

A **secretion** produced by the liver, bile is a yellow-greenish fluid of bitter taste. It is made up of water that contains many dissolved organic and inorganic substances: it has several **bile acids**, **cholesterol**, some minerals and pigments, such as **bilirubin**, a product of digested hemoglobin of red cells that give the secretion its name as well as its coloration. The digestive function of bile is very important, because it eases the digestion of fats contained in food. Some of the elements in bile act upon fats, causing their emulsion, as detergents do, so that the action of enzymes for digestion becomes easier and more efficient.

FUNCTION OF GALLBLADDER AND BILE DUCTS

GALLBLADDER AND BILE DUCTS

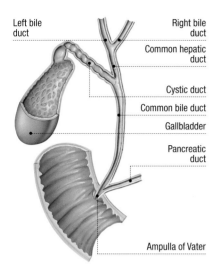

Left bile duct

Right bile duct

Common hepatic duct

Cystic duct

Common bile duct

Gallbladder

Pancreatic duct

Ampulla of Vater

The bile produced by the liver is transported by a series of ducts that take the secretion first to the gallbladder, a **hollow organ** in the shape of a sac, and then to the first portion of the small intestine, where it performs its digestive action. The production of bile is constant, but this secretion is only necessary after eating. During fasting periods, bile coming from the liver through the **bile ducts** alters its course and goes to the gallbladder, where it accumulates and concentrates. During digestion, some hormones produced by the intestine act upon the gallbladder, and make it contract and push out its contents. At the same time, a valve that regulates the communication between the bile ducts and the intestine opens, and the bile is poured into the duodenum.

GALLBLADDER ACTIVITY

Fasting

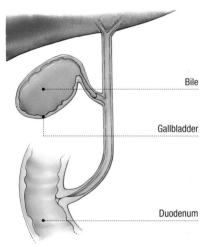

Bile

Gallbladder

Duodenum

During digestion

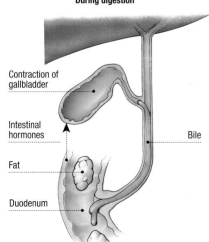

Contraction of gallbladder

Intestinal hormones

Fat

Bile

Duodenum

FUNCTION OF THE PANCREAS

The pancreas is considered **part of the digestive tract**, because, among other functions, it produces a secretion, **pancreatic juice**, essential for digesting food in the small intestine. Inside the organ are many pancreatic acini, some tiny glandular structures made up of only one layer of cells located around a central lumen. These cells pour their secretion into some canaliculi that converge and form ducts through which bile flows into the first portion of the small intestine. The **pancreatic juice** has several **enzymes** that act upon the protein, fats, and carbohydrates, breaking them down to their basic components to facilitate their intestinal absorption.

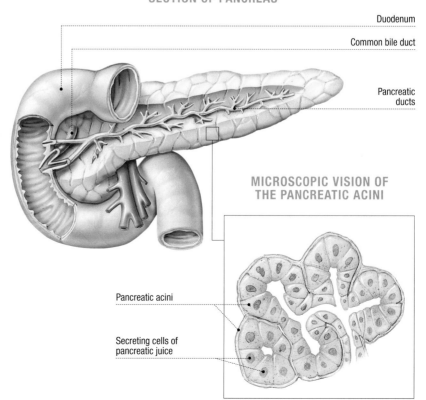

The organs involved in digestion need a large supply of blood, which is why it is necessary to avoid strenuous exercise after a big meal.

SECTION OF PANCREAS

Duodenum

Common bile duct

Pancreatic ducts

MICROSCOPIC VISION OF THE PANCREATIC ACINI

Pancreatic acini

Secreting cells of pancreatic juice

NUTRITION AND METABOLISM

The human body requires the **periodic supply** of a series of basic substances needed for **tissue formation**, for **obtaining the energy** that is needed, for performing its physiological activities, and for regulating metabolism. Such substances, present in different proportions in the foods we eat daily, are the **nutrients**.

NUTRIENTS

Life depends on a continuous exchange of matter and energy, **matter** and **energy** that the body can only obtain from products supplied in foods. But the foods we eat must be subjected to several physical and chemical processes during their passage in the digestive tube to be well utilized: they need to be fragmented into **small particles**, of small enough dimensions that allow them to go through the intestinal walls and into the blood to be distributed all over the body. These small particles, obtained as final products of digestion (**nutrients**), are of varied chemical composition and in various proportions constitute the human body. They are classified in six groups: proteins, carbohydrates, fats, minerals, vitamins, and water.

CHEMICAL COMPOSITION OF THE HUMAN BODY

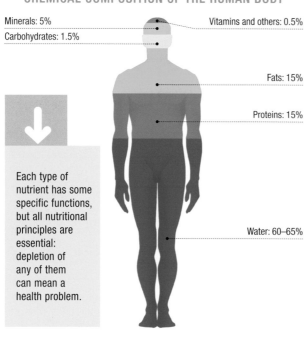

Minerals: 5%

Carbohydrates: 1.5%

Vitamins and others: 0.5%

Fats: 15%

Proteins: 15%

Water: 60–65%

Each type of nutrient has some specific functions, but all nutritional principles are essential: depletion of any of them can mean a health problem.

TYPES OF NUTRIENTS

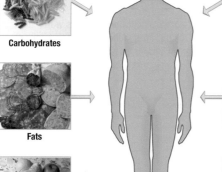

Carbohydrates

Proteins

Fats

Minerals

Vitamins

Water

FUNCTIONS OF NUTRIENTS

The body uses each type of a nutrient in a different way, but generally, it is considered that as a whole, nutrients have three types of functions.

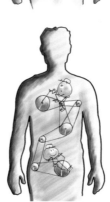

Structural Function

They are used for construction and regeneration of tissues and organs. Proteins and some minerals are used this way.

Energy Function

They are used for obtaining the necessary energy for metabolic chemical reactions that constitute the basis for life, for retaining body heat, for the development of mechanical actions such as muscular contractions, and for many other purposes. Carbohydrates and fats, and secondly, proteins, are used for this purpose.

Regulatory Function

They are used as elements that modulate metabolic chemical reactions and the activity of various organs. Several minerals and vitamins are used for this purpose.

WATER, A VITAL ELEMENT

PROPORTION OF ORGANIC WATER

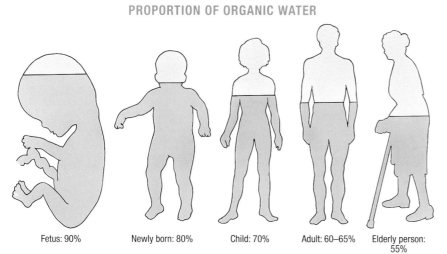

Fetus: 90% Newly born: 80% Child: 70% Adult: 60–65% Elderly person: 55%

Water is the **main component** for human beings and for all living organisms; it is an essential element for life both in terms of quantity and quality. It is not only the largest component of our bodies but also **essential**, because all the chemical reactions necessary for living occur in an aqueous environment. Water is inside all cells (**intracellular fluid**), in between the cells of the various tissues (**intercellular fluid**), and in some body compartments (**extra cellular fluid**), because it is part of blood, the lymph, and organic secretions.

Over half the body mass in humans consists of water, although the percentage decreases throughout life.

WATER BALANCE OF THE ADULT BODY

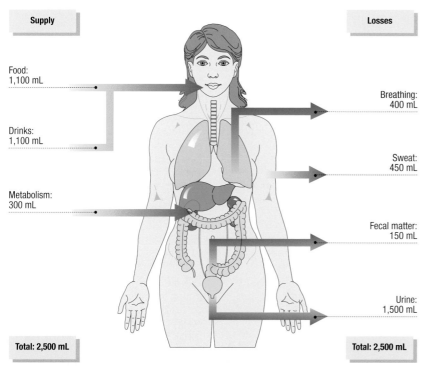

Supply

Food: 1,100 mL

Drinks: 1,100 mL

Metabolism: 300 mL

Total: 2,500 mL

Losses

Breathing: 400 mL

Sweat: 450 mL

Fecal matter: 150 mL

Urine: 1,500 mL

Total: 2,500 mL

WATER MOLECULE

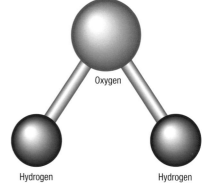

Oxygen

Hydrogen   Hydrogen

WATER NEEDS

The body loses water constantly through various ways: **through waste**, with urine and fecal matter; through the skin, with **sweat**; and through the lungs, with **breathing**. The chemical reactions that take place in the body from the metabolism of carbohydrates, proteins, and fats produce **endogenous water**, about 300 mL a day in the adult, but that amount is not enough to replace what has been lost. Therefore, it is necessary to supply the difference and that can only be achieved with food. **Exogenous water** is provided through drinks, made up mainly of water, and also by food that contains water in smaller or larger proportions.

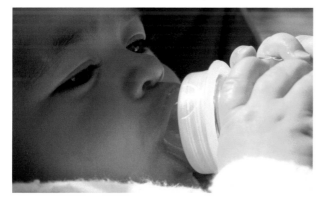

If water losses are not replenished, dehydration can occur, and, in extreme cases, death can occur.

 Without drinking and eating, a person can only live for about a week, or a maximum of 10 days.

CARBOHYDRATES, SOURCE OF ENERGY

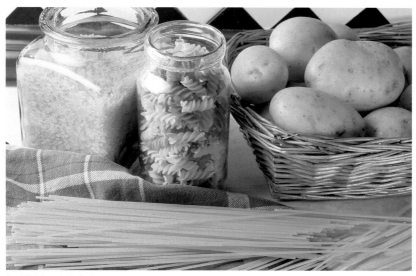

Food rich in carbohydrates.

These nutrients are also called **sugars**, and although they form part of several structures in the body, they especially have an **energetic function**, because the body uses them for obtaining the necessary energy to perform chemical reactions and several biological functions. They are present in various proportions, in almost all foods, especially **vegetables**: the richest ones are cereals and their derivatives, legumes, tubercles, and fruits. Meanwhile common sugar, honey, and all sweets are only made up of carbohydrates.

TYPES OF CARBOHYDRATES

All carbohydrates are made up of **carbon**, **oxygen**, and **hydrogen** atoms, and they receive that name because each carbon atom is linked to an atom of oxygen and two atoms of hydrogen, in the same proportion present in the molecule of water (H_2O). Several kinds can be identified according to their chemical structure and their basic units, called **saccharides**. **Simple carbohydrates** are also called **sugars**, because they have a sweet taste. They may be made up of only one unit and then they are called **monosaccharides**, as is the case of **glucose**, **fructose** (sugar in fruit), and **galactose**. Or they can be made up of two units, in which case they are called **disaccharides**, for example **saccharose** or **sucrose** (ordinary sugar, made up of a glucose molecule and a fructose one), **lactose** (sugar in milk, made up of a glucose molecule and a galactose one), and **maltose** (made up of two galactose molecules). However, **complex carbohydrates**, also called **polysaccharides**, are made up of several simple units linked in long chains, as happens with **starches** or **feculae**, present in vegetables, and in the **glycogen** of animal organisms.

CHEMICAL FORMULA FOR CARBOHYDRATES

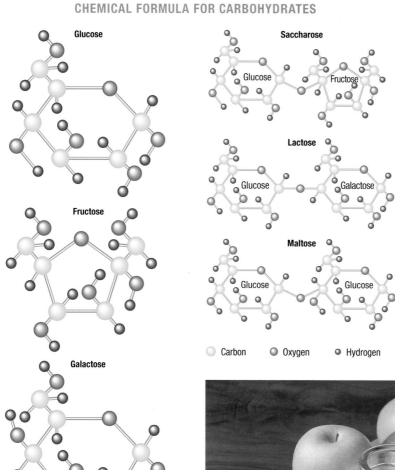

Glucose

Fructose

Galactose

Saccharose
Glucose — Fructose

Lactose
Glucose — Galactose

Maltose
Glucose — Glucose

○ Carbon ● Oxygen ● Hydrogen

○ Carbon ● Oxygen ● Hydrogen

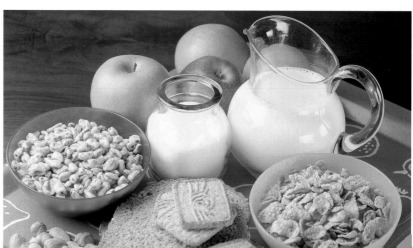

Introduction

A Perfect
Machine

Skin

Digestive
System

Nutrition

Respiratory
System

Circulatory
System and
Blood

Nervous
System

Musculoskeletal
System

Urinary
System

Endocrine
System

Immune
System

The Senses

Genetics

Reproductive
System

Human
Development

Index

CONTENT OF CARBOHYDRATES
(Per 100 grams of food)

Sugar	100 g
Honey	77 g
Rice	77 g
Flour	75 g
Pastas	73 g
Cookies	73 g
Jam	70 g
Confections	60 g
White bread	55 g
Banana	21 g
Boiled potato	20 g

GLUCOSE

The cells in our bodies can only use one carbohydrate as a source of energy: glucose. Glucose molecules, absorbed in the intestine after the digestion of complex carbohydrates or when released by the liver after the transformation of other monosaccharides, travel through the body in the bloodstream and are caught by the cells, inside of which they are subjected to a chemical process of combustion that involves the release of energy.

Glucose is so important that when blood tests are made, you always measure its concentration, called glycemia or "blood sugar," because it is an essential indicator of our health.

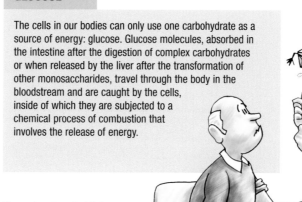

DIGESTION AND ABSORPTION OF CARBOHYDRATES

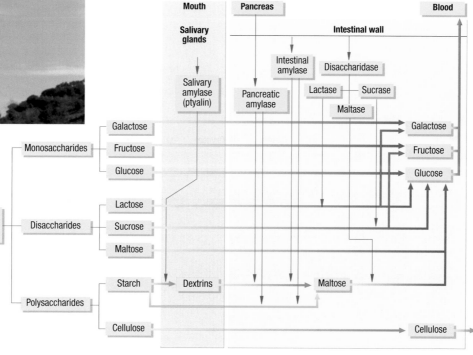

Intracellular combustion of glucose releases approximately 4 kilocalories per gram.

Most of the carbohydrates present in food are disaccharides and polysaccharides, but only monosaccharides, of very small dimensions, can go through the walls of the digestive system. So, to be absorbed, almost all carbohydrates must first be digested, that is to say, **broken down into their basic units**. This happens especially inside the small intestine due to the action of **specific** enzymes like **amylase**, which break the oxygen links and release monosaccharide molecules. Finally in the digestive process, glucose, fructose, and galactose molecules are absorbed. These molecules are taken to the liver, where fructose and galactose are turned into glucose, which is released into the bloodstream to be distributed throughout the body and used as fuel by the cells.

CHEMICAL FORMULA OF CARBOHYDRATES

Mouth — Salivary glands — Salivary amylase (ptyalin)

Pancreas — Pancreatic amylase

Intestinal wall — Intestinal amylase — Disaccharidase — Lactase — Sucrase — Maltase

Blood

Carbo-hydrates

Monosaccharides: Galactose, Fructose, Glucose

Disaccharides: Lactose, Sucrose, Maltose

Polysaccharides: Starch → Dextrins → Maltose, Cellulose

Galactose, Fructose, Glucose, Maltose, Cellulose

PROTEINS: BUILDING MATERIALS

The proteins are the **basic components of the body**, essential for the formation and the development of tissues. They are the building blocks used for making living matter. There are many different proteins in the body, and whereas some of them are structural such as the ones making up cellular walls, muscles, and the framework that supports the organs, others have different functions: **enzymes** involved in metabolism are proteins; **antibodies**, produced by the immune system to protect us from infections; **hormones**; and many other compounds. They can also be used as a source of energy, but it is an extra function. Almost all foods have proteins, although in different proportions and quality: the richest are meats, fish, eggs, milk and some milk by-products, legumes, dry fruits, and cereals and their derivatives.

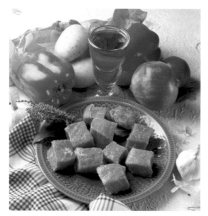

Foods high in proteins.

CHEMICAL FORMULA FOR PROTEINS

Diagram of a tripeptide

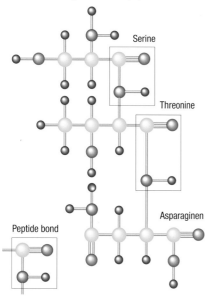

Serine

Threonine

Asparaginen

Peptide bond

Diagram of some amino acids

Serine

Threonine

Asparaginen

- Carbon
- Oxygen
- Hydrogen
- Nitrogen

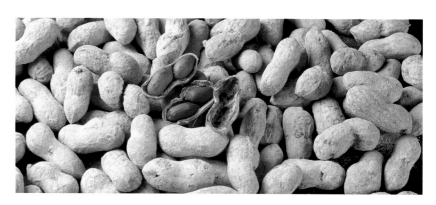

PROTEIN CONTENT (for 100 grams of food)

Parmesan cheese	34 g	Chicken meat	21 g
Soybean	34 g	Ox meat	20.5 g
Turkey meat	32 g	Almonds	20 g
Peanuts	24 g	Hake	17 g
Lentils	24 g	Hazelnut	14 g
Rabbit meat	22 g	Whole egg	13 g
Peas	22 g	Cow's milk	3.5 g

CHEMICAL STRUCTURE OF PROTEINS

Proteins are basically made up of the combination of **carbon**, **oxygen**, **hydrogen**, and **nitrogen** atoms, to which, at times, other chemicals are added. They are made up of a series of subunits: the **amino acids** joined one to another by some special links that form long or short chains. When there are a few units, we speak of **peptides**. Their designation depends on the number of amino acids, for example, dipeptides or tripeptides. When the chains are made up of many amino acids, they are called polypeptides. Some proteins have over a thousand amino acids.

 Approximately 80% of the dry weight of cells corresponds to proteins.

TYPES OF AMINO ACIDS

All proteins in nature are made up of a combination of only 20 different amino acids; each one has its own chemical structure: amino acids are something like the letters of the alphabet with which you form thousands and thousands of different words. To form its own proteins, the human body needs to have all amino acids at its disposal. Actually, the body can synthesize some, the **nonessential amino acids**, but can only obtain others, **essential amino acids**, through food. That is why it is so important to eat a variety of foods that provide all types of amino acids and especially essential amino acids, which are present in products of animal origin.

ESSENTIAL AMINO ACIDS	NONESSENTIAL AMINO ACIDS
Arginine*	Glutamic acid
Phenylalanine	Alanine
Histidine*	Asparagine
Isoleucine	Cysteine
Leucine	Cystine
Lysine	Glycine
Methionine	Hydroxyproline
Threonine	Proline
Tryptophan	Serine
Valine	Tyrosine

*essential for children

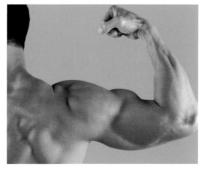

Intracellular combustion of proteins releases approximately 4 kilocalories per gram.

The combination of various foods increases their biological value, because the body obtains several amino acids with which to make its own proteins.

DIGESTION AND ABSORPTION OF PROTEINS

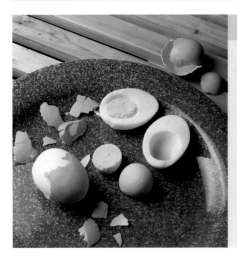

QUALITY PROTEINS

Not all the proteins we eat have the same biological value. Proteins high in essential amino acids are considered better quality, and the body has to obtain them through foods. Proteins of higher biological value are those of hen eggs, which are taken as a "pattern" to classify the rest. According to this criterion, it is considered that proteins of animal origin have a higher biological value than proteins of plant origin.

The digestion of proteins contained in foods starts in the stomach through the action of the gastric juice. Hydrochloric acid produced by the mucosa of the stomach activates an enzyme called **pepsin**, which acts upon proteins and destroys some links, breaking them down and releasing polypeptide chains of smaller dimensions. When food goes to the small intestine, some enzymes produced by the pancreas release amino acids, dipeptides, and tripeptides, which are absorbed by cells in the intestinal wall. The breaking down is completed inside these cells, in such a way that only free amino acids are released into the bloodstream. Then, after being distributed throughout the body, the various amino acids combine with each other to form organic proteins.

Eggs are one the most complete foods and should not be absent from our diets, because they have maximum quality proteins and also fats, minerals, and vitamins.

DIAGRAM OF DIGESTION AND ABSORPTION OF PROTEINS

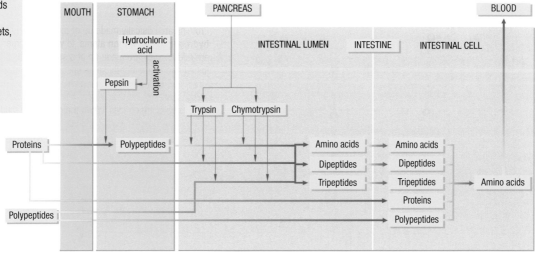

Introduction

A Perfect Machine

Skin

Digestive System

Nutrition

Respiratory System

Circulatory System and Blood

Nervous System

Musculoskeletal System

Urinary System

Endocrine System

Immune System

The Senses

Genetics

Reproductive System

Human Development

Index

FATS: CONCENTRATED ENERGY

Also called **lipids**, fats are the most energy-rich nutrients. The body uses the fats in the foods we eat to **obtain energy**, and, conversely, it stores any excess energy as fats after using other nutrients. Fats are present in almost all foods, although in different proportions. They are the only ingredient in **oils** and the main ingredient in **butter** and **margarine**. Meats, fowl, some fish, milk and its derivates, eggs, and dried fruits have lipids in smaller amounts.

Intracellular combustion of fats releases approximately 9 kilocalories per gram.

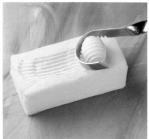

Foods high in fats.

CHEMICAL STRUCTURE OF FATS

Fats are made up of atoms of **carbon**, **oxygen**, and **hydrogen**, combined in such a way that they provide nutrients with a peculiar characteristic: they do not dissolve in water. The most common lipids are **triglycerides**, which are made up of one alcohol molecule called **glycerol** and three molecules of fatty acids. Because there are approximately 40 different **fatty acids**, the possible combinations are numerous. And, fatty acids, formed essentially by a long chain of carbon atoms bonded to other carbon atoms and two hydrogen atoms, can be divided into different types. When carbon atoms are attached to the maximum number of hydrogen atoms possible, it is said that they are saturated, because it is not possible for them to bind with any other hydrogen atom. If they have free bonds, it is said they are **unsaturated**, either **monounsaturated**, when there is one free bond, or **polyunsaturated**, when there are several free bonds.

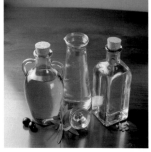
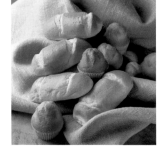

FAT CONTENT (per 100 grams of food)

Oils	100 g	Almonds	54 g
Butter	83 g	French fries	37 g
Margarine	83 g	Chocolate milk	34 g
Mayonnaise	78 g	Cheese	33 g
Bacon	70 g	Milk cream	30 g
Coconut	60 g	Pork	25 g
Hazelnuts	60 g	Ox meat	20 g
Peanuts	60 g	Avocado	16 g
Walnuts	60 g	Duck meat	15 g

CHEMICAL FORMULA OF FATS

Diagram of a triglyceride

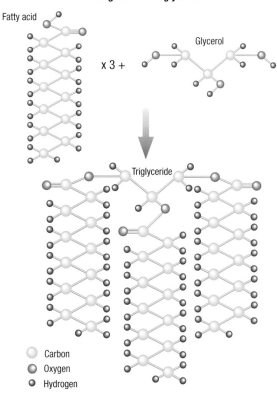

Fatty acid

x 3 +

Glycerol

Triglyceride

○ Carbon
◔ Oxygen
● Hydrogen

Diagram of fatty acids

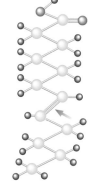
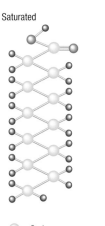
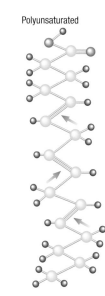

Saturated

Monounsaturated

Polyunsaturated

○ Carbon
◔ Oxygen
● Hydrogen
→ Double bond

DIGESTION AND ABSORPTION OF FATS

CONTENT IN FATTY ACIDS SATURATED AND UNSATURATED

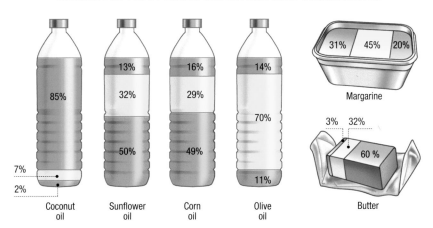

Coconut oil: 85%, 7%, 2%

Sunflower oil: 13%, 32%, 50%

Corn oil: 16%, 29%, 49%

Olive oil: 14%, 70%, 11%

Margarine: 31%, 45%, 20%

Butter: 3%, 32%, 60%

- Polyunsaturated
- Monounsaturated
- Saturated

Fats in foods, after chewing and gastric crushing, arrive in the intestine as small drops that, although tiny, still cannot be processed by digestive enzymes. In the duodenum, **bile** produced from the liver acts upon these droplets and has an emulsifying effect, similar to that of dish soap, breaking them down into microscopic particles called **micelles**. Pancreatic and intestinal enzymes called **lipases** act upon them and release gastric acid so that they can penetrate the intestinal cells, where they regroup and constitute particles called chylomicrons, which are soluble in organic fluids. **Chylomicrons** travel to the lymph vessels of the intestinal villi and via lymph circulation get to the bloodstream so that they can be distributed throughout the body.

ANIMAL AND PLANT FATS

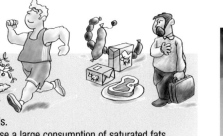

There is a very important difference between fats of animal and plant origin: the former are high in saturated fatty acids, whereas the latter have a larger proportion of unsaturated fatty acids.

This difference is closely related to health, because a large consumption of saturated fats of animal origin predisposes one to **heart disease**. Unsaturated fats, of plant origin, have a **protective effect**. Thus, while it is advisable to moderate the consumption of fats to avoid obesity, it is necessary to limit the intake of fats of animal origin.

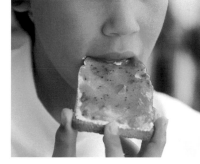

It is still true that chewing well is half of digestion.

Lipids are the nutrients that take the longest to digest. That is why the digestion of foods high in fats, such as fried foods and stews, is slow.

DIAGRAM OF DIGESTION AND ABSORPTION OF FATS

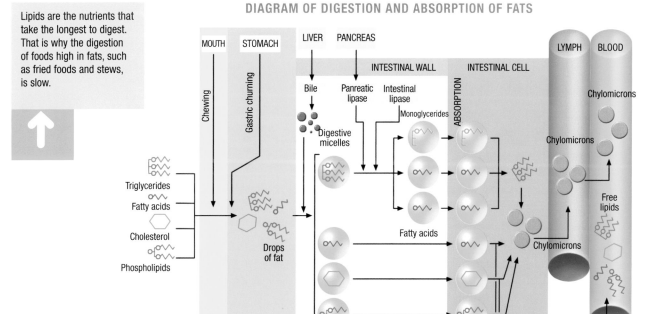

Introduction

A Perfect Machine

Skin

Digestive System

Nutrition

Respiratory System

Circulatory System and Blood

Nervous System

Musculoskeletal System

Urinary System

Endocrine System

Immune System

The Senses

Genetics

Reproductive System

Human Development

Index

MINERALS

Minerals are inorganic elements considered basic nutrients, because a regular supply of them is needed for the formation and working of the body. Some have a **plastic function**, because they are part of organic structures; such is the case with calcium contained in bones and teeth. Others, however, develop a **regulatory function** because they are part of enzymes and hormones taking part in numerous metabolic processes. These nutrients are especially essential during childhood and adolescence, because, during this time, the body is in the middle of **growing** and **developing**, although minerals continue to be necessary throughout life to replenish the continuous losses resulting from elimination of waste and secretions. Practically all foods have minerals, but the requirements of these nutrients can only be met by eating a variety of foods.

→ Overall, minerals represent approximately 5% of body weight.

TYPES OF MINERALS

In nutrition, minerals are classified into two groups according to the body's everyday requirements of them. Some are included in the group of **macronutrients**, because their presence in the body is important, and they are needed regularly through food. Among these, the most important are calcium, iron, phosphorus, sodium, potassium, and magnesium. Others, however, are included in the group of **micronutrients**, also called **oligoelements**, because the body's content of them is very small, and only a minimum regular supply through foods is needed to meet the requirements. In this group, we find selenium, fluoride, iodine, manganese, copper, molybdenum, zinc, chrome, cobalt, nickel, and vanadium.

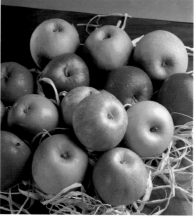

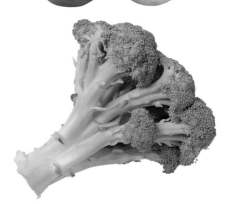

Fruits and vegetables are excellent sources of minerals and thus should be part of our daily diet.

ROLES OF THE MOST IMPORTANT MINERALS

MINERAL	ROLES
Calcium	It is the most plentiful mineral in our bodies. It is part of the bone structure; it has a regulatory action on many organic processes; and it takes part in the transmission of nerve impulses, the mechanism of muscular contraction, and blood clotting.
Phosphorus	It is part of the bone structure and teeth; it is a component of the cellular membranes, and it makes up the chromosomes; it takes part in processes for obtaining energy, the mechanism of muscular contraction, and several metabolic reactions.
Iron	It is a basic component of the hemoglobin of red cells and of several enzymes that take part in metabolism.
Sodium	It takes part in the regulation of body fluids and blood pressure, as well as the transmission of nerve impulses, the heartbeat, and the mechanism of muscular contraction.
Potassium	It acts together with sodium in the transmission of nerve impulses and the regulation of body fluids. It also takes part in the metabolism of carbohydrates and proteins.
Iodine	It is part of the hormones produced by the thyroid gland that regulate the general metabolism and have an important role in the growing process and the maturation of the nerve system.
Fluoride	It is a component in bones and in teeth, providing resistance and protection against cavities.
Magnesium	It is a component in bones; it takes part in the activation of intracellular enzymes and in the transmission of impulses in muscle tissue.

Milk is one of the most complete foods in terms of minerals and vitamins.

VITAMINS

Vitamins are chemical substances of varied nature, but they have something very important in common: the body needs to incorporate them through foods, even if in small amounts, to guarantee the body's performance. Vitamins have a **regulatory** **function**, because they take part in several essential metabolic processes, and, if there is not enough supply, there is a **vitamin deficiency**, which causes specific organic disorders, depending on the vitamin. Although each vitamin has a specific name, letters of the alphabet and subindexes are generally used to designate the various vitamins. These designations were given as vitamins were being discovered, when their chemical formula was still unknown.

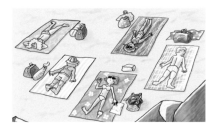

Unlike other vitamins, vitamin D can be synthesized in the body. This happens in the skin due to stimulation by exposure to sun.

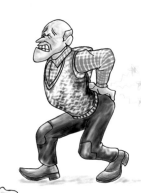

Carrots are high in vitamin A, or retinol, which is very beneficial for eyesight.

TYPES OF VITAMINS

Altogether, 13 vitamins are known, and they are classified in two groups, not according to their function but to their soluble properties. One group is composed of the water solubles (**hydro soluble**), such as vitamin C and the vitamin B complex. One characteristic these vitamins have is that because they are soluble in water, if there is an overdose, they are eliminated by the kidneys through urine. The other group corresponds to **lipo soluble vitamins** or fat solubles, such as vitamins A, D, E, and K. These vitamins can only be found in foods having a certain amount of fats, and their absorption requires the presence of fats. Because they tend to build up in fat tissues, if there is an excessive intake, they stay in the body, causing a condition called **hypervitaminosis**, with specific manifestations, depending on the vitamin.

ROLES AND SOURCES OF THE MAIN VITAMINS

VITAMIN	ROLES	SOURCES
Vitamin A Retinol	Takes part in the vision mechanism, allowing the eyes to adapt to semidarkness, and it takes part in the regeneration of epithelial tissues during growth and reproduction	Milk; milk products; liver; egg yolk; oily fish; vegetables high in carotene, such as carrots, sweet potatoes, squash, and green leafy vegetables
Vitamin B_1 Thiamine	Involved in metabolizing carbohydrates, in several biological reactions, in the stimulation of peripheral nerves, and in heart and intestinal activity	Whole-wheat cereal and derivates, yeast, milk, egg, pork, dried fruits, legumes, and vegetables in general
Vitamin B_2 Riboflavin	Involved in breathing and intracellular oxidation, it takes part in the metabolism of hemoglobin, and acts as a coenzyme in the metabolism of carbohydrates, proteins, and fats	Kidney, liver, yeast, milk and milk products, egg, dried fruits, whole-wheat cereals, and vegetables
Vitamin B_3 Niacin	Takes part in the metabolism of carbohydrates, proteins, and fats, and the synthesis of several substances	Red meat, entrails, fish, fowls, legumes, milk and milk products, whole-wheat cereals and derivates
Vitamin B_5 Pantothenic Acid	Takes part in the metabolism of carbohydrates, proteins, and fats, and also in chemical reactions of several phenomena	Present in almost all foods
Vitamin B_6 Pyridoxine	Takes part in the metabolism of proteins, in blood formation, and in the activity in the nervous system	Yeast, red meats, fish, fowls, milk, legumes, soy, whole-wheat cereals and derivates, dried fruits, fresh fruits
Vitamin B_9 Folic acid	Takes part in the maturation of red cells and in the process of cellular division, and it is essential for the formation of new tissues during growth	Liver, legumes, cereals, soy, milk, meat, dried fruits, green leafy vegetables, fresh fruit
Vitamin B_{12} Cyanocobalamin	Involved in the metabolism of carbohydrates, proteins and fats, in red cell maturation in blood, in nuclear acid synthesis and the activity of the nervous system	Liver, kidney, meat, fish, milk and milk products, eggs; absent in plant origin foods
Vitamin C Ascorbic acid	Involved in intracellular metabolism, it plays a protective role on the skin and mucosa; it takes part in the production of some hormones, and aids iron absorption in the intestine	Fruits (citric, kiwi, pineapple, berries) and fresh vegetables (pepper, broccoli, cabbage, watercress, Swiss chard, potatoes, squash)
Vitamin D Calciferol	Involved in the regulation of calcium and phosphorus metabolism, it is important for bones; it takes part in muscular activity, essential for growing	Liver, seafood, meat, milk and milk products, eggs; it is produced in the skin under the influence of the sun
Vitamin E Tocopherol	Has an antioxidant action and takes part in maintaining cell membranes	Eggs, seed oils, legumes, vegetables, dried fruits
Vitamin K Menaquinone	Essential in the production of substances promoting clotting, its presence in the blood is fundamental for preventing blood loss	Liver, kidney, vegetables, and fruits; it is synthesized by bacteria of the intestinal flora

Vitamin D or calciferol is essential for healthy bones

Vitamin K is involved in the blood clotting mechanisms.

Introduction

A Perfect Machine

Skin

Digestive System

Nutrition

Respiratory System

Circulatory System and Blood

Nervous System

Musculoskeletal System

Urinary System

Endocrine System

Immune System

The Senses

Genetics

Reproductive System

Human Development

Index

THE RESPIRATORY SYSTEM

The respiratory system's objective is the **gas exchange** between the body and the outside air, and it has two supplementary functions: on one hand, it is in charge of **obtaining oxygen**, a vital element for the metabolic activity in all the cells in our body; on the other hand, it is responsible for the **elimination of carbon dioxide**, a waste product whose buildup in the body is toxic.

COMPONENTS OF THE RESPIRATORY SYSTEM

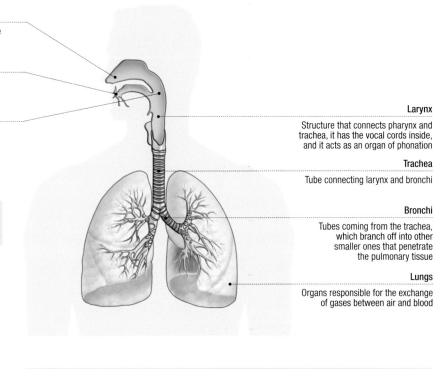

Nose
Main access way of air into the body; it conditions the air so that it gets to the lungs in an optimal state

Mouth
Secondary way for air to go in and out; it is considered part of the digestive system

Pharynx
Region located behind the nostrils and the mouth;, it is part of both the respiratory and digestive systems, because it directs air to the larynx and food to the stomach.

Larynx
Structure that connects pharynx and trachea, it has the vocal cords inside, and it acts as an organ of phonation

Trachea
Tube connecting larynx and bronchi

Bronchi
Tubes coming from the trachea, which branch off into other smaller ones that penetrate the pulmonary tissue

Lungs
Organs responsible for the exchange of gases between air and blood

AIR PASSAGES

Air must follow a path made up of a series of **air passages** to travel from the outside into the lungs and from the lungs back to the outside. Traditionally, airways are divided into two parts: **upper respiratory system**, made up of the nose and the pharynx, which are connected to the upper part of the digestive system and even share some structures with it, and **lower respiratory system**, made up of the larynx, the trachea, and the bronchi, which are organs belonging exclusively to the respiratory system.

Breathing is a vital function, because the suspension of this activity will cause death.

LUNGS

The lungs are two **spongy organs**, in the shape of a cone and divided into several **lobules** that are located inside the chest cavity. They are covered by a double membrane called **pleura** and are separated from the abdominal cavity by a powerful flat muscle, the **diaphragm**, which is mainly responsible for breathing movements. Bronchi subdivide into **bronchioles**, which subdivide into 16 generations. These small bronchioles open into **alveoli**, tiny sacs with thin walls and surrounded by capillaries where the gas exchange between air and blood occurs.

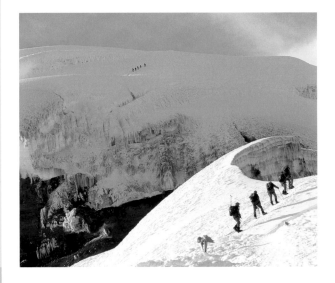

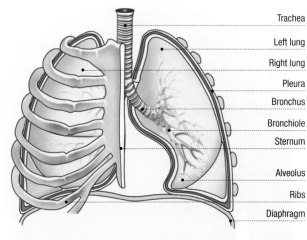

Trachea
Left lung
Right lung
Pleura
Bronchus
Bronchiole
Sternum
Alveolus
Ribs
Diaphragm

Introduction

A Perfect Machine

Skin

Digestive System

Nutrition

Respiratory System

Circulatory System and Blood

Nervous System

Musculoskeletal System

Urinary System

Endocrine System

Immune System

The Senses

Genetics

Reproductive System

Human Development

Index

BREATHING MECHANISM

Inspiration

Air entry

External intercostals contraction

Lung expansion

Negative pressure in alveoli

Negative pressure in pleural space

Contraction of Diaphragm

Expiration

Air exit

Elastic recoil of lung

External intercostals relaxation

Positive pressure in alveoli

Diaphragm relaxation

BREATHING MOVEMENTS

The air going in and out of the lungs is due to the action of powerful **breathing muscles**, and when they contract and relax in a synchronized way, they alternatively expand and retract the rib cage. The drawing of air from the outside into the lungs, **inhalation**, is done mainly by a contraction of the diaphragm and the external intercostals: the diaphragm flattens and expands the rib cage, while the intercostals raise the lower ribs and increase the thoracic depth. Breathing the air out of the lungs, **exhalation**, is basically a passive mechanism, because they are elastic, and when the inhaling muscles relax and stop their expansion of the rib cage, the lungs tend to return to their normal size, pushing the air out.

NERVOUS REGULATION OF BREATHING

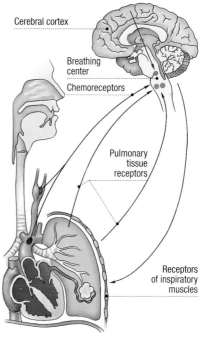

Cerebral cortex

Breathing center

Chemoreceptors

Pulmonary tissue receptors

Receptors of inspiratory muscles

CONTROL OF BREATHING MOVEMENTS

Although breathing movements can be made at will, under normal conditions they happen spontaneously. We do not need to think about it, due to the controlling action of the **nervous breathing center** located in the brain stem, which regulates the frequency and intensity of the inhalations.

This breathing center, formed by three nuclei, receives, on the one hand, stimuli from the cerebral cortex and, on the other hand, from specific receptors distributed in several tissues and organs that can detect chemical parameters, such as the levels of blood gases, the degree of stretching of the pulmonary tissue, or the conditions of the inhaling muscles. When processing all this information, the breathing center determines, automatically, the best rhythm of breathing, according to the needs of each moment.

Breathing is slow when we are at rest and faster when we exercise.

THE ANNOYING HICCUPS

Hiccups happen when for some reason the diaphragm contracts suddenly and does not allow time for the vocal folds in the larynx to separate: the air impacts against the closed vocal cords and generates a characteristic guttural sound. It is almost always due to an untimely stimulus from the nervous breathing center, for example, as a response to an exaggerated distension of the diaphragm caused by a large meal. Different remedies have been suggested, although they do not always work. For example, it can be useful to distract the affected person, although there are some people who think it is more effective to scare the person. Another method is to breathe in without releasing the air for as long as possible, either by holding your breath or by drinking sips of water without breathing.

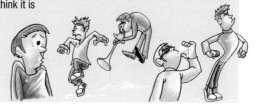

THE NOSE, A NATURAL FILTER

FUNCTIONS OF THE NOSE

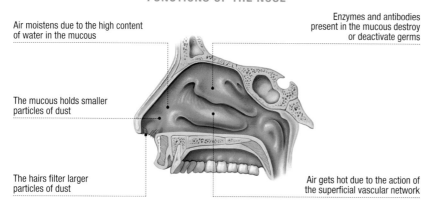

Air moistens due to the high content of water in the mucous

Enzymes and antibodies present in the mucous destroy or deactivate germs

The mucous holds smaller particles of dust

The hairs filter larger particles of dust

Air gets hot due to the action of the superficial vascular network

The nose is the natural air passage to the inside of the body, but it is also in charge of **conditioning** the air we inhale so that it arrives in the lungs in an optimal state. The nose acts as a **filter** for the particles floating in the air, while the high water content of the mucous that covers the nostrils provides the air we inhale with an **optimal degree of humidity**. The large superficial vascular network transports and warms the air in such a way that even in cold weather it reaches an **ideal** and harmless **temperature** before arriving in the lungs.

HYGIENE

It is possible to breathe through the nose or mouth, but ideally it is done through the nose, because the air purifies and acquires the temperature and humidity conditions that are optimal for its arrival in the lungs.

It is not advisable to suppress a sneeze, because they are always beneficial to clean the nose: if you hold in a sneeze, the pressure of the compressed air in the lungs can be harmful to the delicate tissue of these organs.

It is always advisable to cover your nose with a handkerchief when sneezing: the air pushed out releases the nostrils and spreads the germs, many meters, that cause colds. This is a key factor in the spread of the illness.

THE SNEEZE: A PROTECTIVE MECHANISM

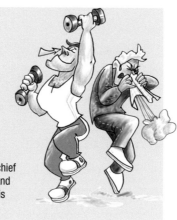

Sneezing is a **reflex action** designed to push out all excess mucus in the nostrils or any impurity that has entered with the inhaled air, in other words, to **clean the nose**. It happens automatically when particles irritate the sensitive nerve endings in the nasal mucosa: dust particles, a foreign body, or an irritant gas. Those stimuli travel through a nerve to the **sneezing center**, located in the brain, and there several orders are generated, which cause a chain reaction.

First, there is a deep inhalation and the lungs fill with air; next, the respiratory muscles contract very hard, which compress the lungs abruptly and form an air current that travels rapidly through the airways. At that moment, the vocal chords open completely to allow the passage of air, and at the same time, the velum (soft palate) lowers to guide it to the nose. The air violently passes through the nostrils and is forced out with a characteristic sound.

SNEEZE MECHANISM

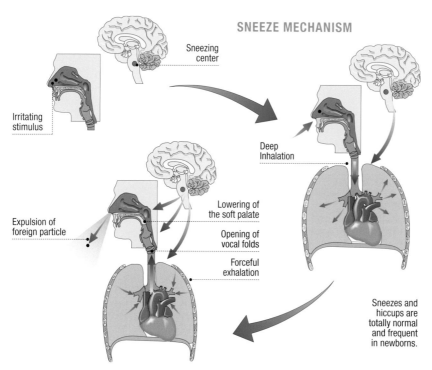

Sneezing center

Irritating stimulus

Deep Inhalation

Lowering of the soft palate

Opening of vocal folds

Forceful exhalation

Expulsion of foreign particle

Sneezes and hiccups are totally normal and frequent in newborns.

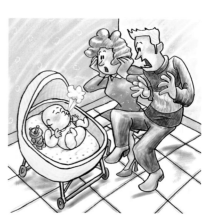

THE PHARYNX: REGULATOR OF AIR AND FOOD

FUNCTIONS OF THE PHARYNX

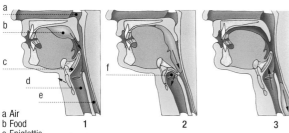

a Air
b Food
c Epiglottis
d Larynx
e Esophagus
f Epiglottis

1   2   3

(**1**) when inhaling, the epiglottis stays up and the air moves to the larynx
(**2**) when swallowing, the epiglottis closes the airway and the food goes to the esophagus
(**3**) the epiglottis raises again, and the air passes again to the larynx

The pharynx is a wide space behind the nostrils and oral cavity that goes inside the neck and ends in the larynx and esophagus. It is part, therefore, of both the respiratory and digestive systems. This **double function** of the pharynx in the passage of air and food is possible due to the **epiglottis**, a cartilage with the shape of a tennis racquet located in the upper part of the larynx and that is usually open. This cartilage allows air communication between the larynx and the outside, but it closes during deglutition and blocks the entry to the larynx, directing the bolus to the stomach.

STRUCTURE OF THE LARYNX

Anterior view
- Epiglottis
- Hyoid bone
- Thyroid cartilage

Postier view
- Hyoid bone
- Epiglottis
- Thyroid cartilage
- Arytenoid cartilage
- Cricoid cartilage

Lateral view
- Epiglottis
- Thyroid cartilage
- Hyoid bone
- Cricoid cartilage

THE LARYNX: VOICE ORGAN

The larynx is made up of a series of **articulated cartilages** that are joined to one another by several muscles, membranes, and ligaments. It is located between the pharynx and the trachea, and is an **unavoidable air passage** during either inhalation or exhalation. But it also has another not less important function: **the production of sounds** that gives us voice. On top of its internal surface, there are two folds on each side, some fibrous ones (vestibular folds or **false vocal chords**) and other fibromuscular ones (true **vocal chords**). They are separated by a slit in the shape of a V, known as **glottis**, and are responsible for the production of sounds.

VOICE PRODUCTION

During exhalation and inhalation, when you are not talking, the **vocal chords** are **relaxed** and stay folded toward the larynx walls, separated by a space, and allowing the free passage of air. However, when you speak, due to the action of muscles that control the larynx cartilages, during exhalation, the **vocal chords tense up** and come closer to the middle line and vibrate when the air from the lungs passes through them. This causes the production of sound, with different tones according to the degree of tension and shape the vocal chords momentarily adopt.

Singing is the art of producing or reproducing melodic sounds with the voice.

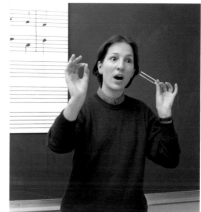

LOCATION OF VOCAL CHORDS

Lateral view
- Arytenoid cartilage
- Vocal folds
- Thyroid cartilage
- Cricoid cartilage

Anterior view
- False vocal chords
- Glottis
- Vocal chords

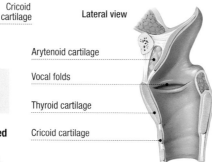
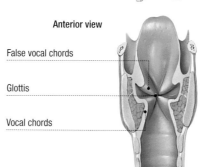

VOICE QUALITY

Pitch: Higher or lower. It depends on the degree of tension of the vocal chords when the sound is produced.

Loudness: It is the volume. It depends on the strength of the air current coming from the lungs, which act as bellows activated by the respiratory muscles.

Timbre: It is particular of each person because it depends on their way of speaking, the shape of the cavities that act as a resonance box (nostrils, paranasal sinuses), and the characteristics of other elements involved in the articulation of sounds (lips, cheeks, teeth, tongue, etc.).

FUNCTION OF THE RESPIRATORY MUCOSA

The **mucosa layer** that covers the inside of the airways is formed primarily of cells whose surface is covered by several **cilia**, similar to tiny eyelashes or mobile filaments. Other cells placed among them are in charge of **secreting mucus**. The mucus forms a viscous film where small solid particles present in the air that have passed through the filter in the upper respiratory tract are trapped. The **coordinated** **movements** of the cilia, in a similar motion to that of the wheat spikes in a field, move the mucus out as if on a conveyor belt. In this way, the mucus flows continuously from the bronchi and the trachea to the throat and goes to the pharynx to be swallowed; we swallow it automatically, almost without noticing.

STRUCTURE OF TRACHEA AND BRONCHI

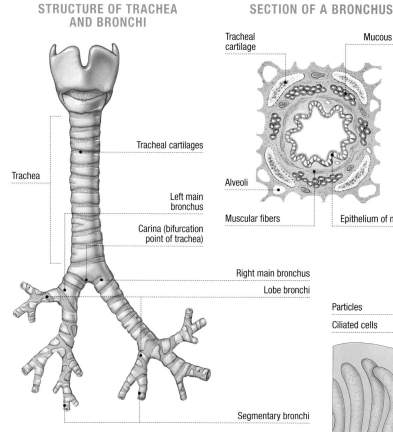

Trachea

Tracheal cartilages

Left main bronchus

Carina (bifurcation point of trachea)

Right main bronchus

Lobe bronchi

Segmentary bronchi

SECTION OF A BRONCHUS

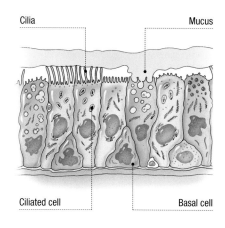

Tracheal cartilage

Mucous glands

Alveoli

Muscular fibers

Epithelium of mucosa

RESPIRATORY MUCOSA

Cilia

Mucus

Ciliated cell

Basal cell

ACTION OF CILIA

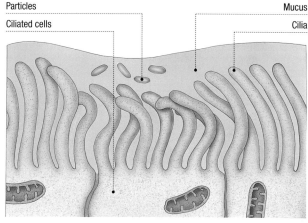

Particles

Mucus

Ciliated cells

Cilia

Tiny particles coming from the outside are trapped in the mucus

Direction of movement

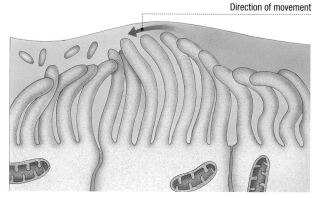

The coordinated movement of cilia moves the mucus toward the pharynx

A persistent or repetitive cough, or one accompanied by pain is a symptom of respiratory disease: you should consult a doctor to discover its origin and to receive the appropriate treatment.

The lungs have millions of alveoli, which, although tiny, form a surface for gas exchange of approximately 150 m^2.

HYGIENE

Coughing pushes out many saliva droplets that can contain germs responsible for infectious diseases. In order not to contribute to spreading these germs, it is advisable to cover your mouth with your hand when coughing or if it is a productive cough, use a tissue.

COUGHING

Coughing is a reflex that has a defensive function. Although it can be done at will, it usually occurs automatically when there is some irritation or obstruction in the larynx, trachea, or bronchi. Its goal is to eliminate all obstacles to the passage of air through the airways. The reflex is controlled by a nerve center located in the medulla, and it starts when there is any irritant, chemical, or mechanical stimuli in the mucosa of the lower airways, such as the inhalation of dust, smoke or gases, an inflammatory process, a foreign body, secretion buildup, etc. First, there is a deep inhalation and immediately after, the respiratory muscles contract tightly. At first the vocal chords stay closed, preventing the air from coming out. Next, the vocal chords open abruptly, allowing a violent air current to go through the respiratory tract, dragging out irritants, secretions, or any foreign bodies.

Introduction

A Perfect Machine

Skin

Digestive System

Nutrition

Respiratory System

Circulatory System and Blood

Nervous System

Musculoskeletal System

Urinary System

Endocrine System

Immune System

The Senses

Genetics

Reproductive System

Human Development

Index

COUGH MECHANISM

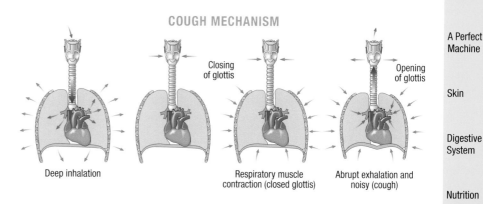

Deep inhalation

Closing of glottis

Respiratory muscle contraction (closed glottis)

Opening of glottis

Abrupt exhalation and noisy (cough)

THE FUNCTIONAL UNIT OF LUNGS

After several branches, bronchi are divided into very thin ducts, **bronchioles**, which have several **alveoli** at their ends, microscopic sacs with very thin walls, because they are made up of only one layer of cells. These tiny bags that fill up with air in each inhalation and empty in each exhalation are surrounded by many **capillary vessels** with very thin walls where blood constantly circulates. It is precisely in between these two elements, alveoli and capillaries, where the main activity of the lungs takes place: the gas exchange between air and blood.

MECHANISM OF GAS EXCHANGE

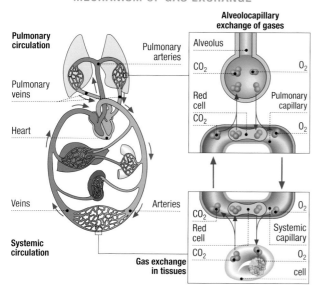

Pulmonary circulation

Pulmonary arteries

Pulmonary veins

Heart

Veins

Arteries

Systemic circulation

Alveolocapillary exchange of gases

Alveolus

CO_2 — O_2

Red cell

CO_2 — O_2

Pulmonary capillary

CO_2 — O_2

Red cell

CO_2 — O_2

Systemic capillary

cell

Gas exchange in tissues

BRONCHIOLES AND ALVEOLI

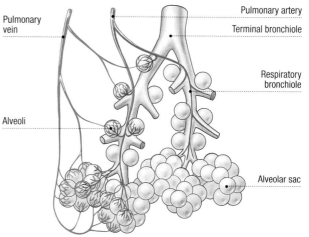

Pulmonary vein

Alveoli

Pulmonary artery

Terminal bronchiole

Respiratory bronchiole

Alveolar sac

GAS EXCHANGE

The molecules of oxygen (O_2) and carbon dioxide (CO_2) circulate in the blood bound to **the hemoglobin** of the red cells, which transports these gases throughout the body. In their circulation, the red cells move to the lungs where there is a gas exchange with the air arriving at the alveoli when inhaling. This is a simple **diffusion mechanism**. Oxygen goes from the air to the blood, while carbon dioxide goes from inside the capillaries into the alveoli, to be breathed out with exhalation. After passing through the lungs, the blood high in oxygen and low in carbon dioxide, continues its path and driven by the heart moves by means of the systemic circulation to the capillaries in various tissues. There, also due to a diffusion mechanism, oxygen goes from the blood to the cells and carbon dioxide goes from the cells to the blood. And the blood, low in oxygen and full of carbon dioxide, continues its path until it reaches the lungs again. There a new gas exchange occurs in a cycle that goes on endlessly throughout life.

OXYGEN, VITAL GAS

The human body needs constant gas exchange with the atmosphere: on the one hand, it needs to integrate **oxygen**, an essential element for cellular activity used as a fuel to obtain the energy used in metabolic reactions; on the other hand, it has to get rid of **carbon dioxide** produced as residue of metabolism, because it is toxic if it builds up in the body. Cells need a **constant supply** of oxygen, otherwise they cannot work. Some cells, neurons for example, can hardly last a few minutes without oxygen.

THE CIRCULATORY SYSTEM

The circulatory system is also called the **cardio-vascular system**, because it is formed by the **heart** and a complex network of **blood vessels**. Its function is to carry blood continuously to all tissues in the body. Blood provides the tissues with **oxygen** and **nutrients** needed for functioning, and it picks up **metabolic residues** for transport to the organs in charge of eliminating them.

MAIN COMPONENTS OF THE CIRCULATORY SYSTEM

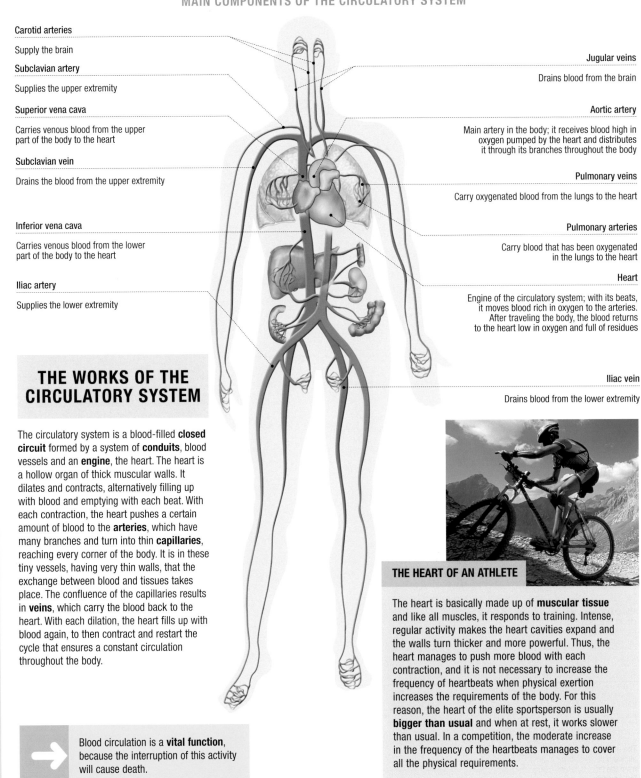

Carotid arteries

Supply the brain

Subclavian artery

Supplies the upper extremity

Superior vena cava

Carries venous blood from the upper part of the body to the heart

Subclavian vein

Drains the blood from the upper extremity

Inferior vena cava

Carries venous blood from the lower part of the body to the heart

Iliac artery

Supplies the lower extremity

Jugular veins

Drains blood from the brain

Aortic artery

Main artery in the body; it receives blood high in oxygen pumped by the heart and distributes it through its branches throughout the body

Pulmonary veins

Carry oxygenated blood from the lungs to the heart

Pulmonary arteries

Carry blood that has been oxygenated in the lungs to the heart

Heart

Engine of the circulatory system; with its beats, it moves blood rich in oxygen to the arteries. After traveling the body, the blood returns to the heart low in oxygen and full of residues

Iliac vein

Drains blood from the lower extremity

THE WORKS OF THE CIRCULATORY SYSTEM

The circulatory system is a blood-filled **closed circuit** formed by a system of **conduits**, blood vessels and an **engine**, the heart. The heart is a hollow organ of thick muscular walls. It dilates and contracts, alternatively filling up with blood and emptying with each beat. With each contraction, the heart pushes a certain amount of blood to the **arteries**, which have many branches and turn into thin **capillaries**, reaching every corner of the body. It is in these tiny vessels, having very thin walls, that the exchange between blood and tissues takes place. The confluence of the capillaries results in **veins**, which carry the blood back to the heart. With each dilation, the heart fills up with blood again, to then contract and restart the cycle that ensures a constant circulation throughout the body.

→ Blood circulation is a **vital function**, because the interruption of this activity will cause death.

THE HEART OF AN ATHLETE

The heart is basically made up of **muscular tissue** and like all muscles, it responds to training. Intense, regular activity makes the heart cavities expand and the walls turn thicker and more powerful. Thus, the heart manages to push more blood with each contraction, and it is not necessary to increase the frequency of heartbeats when physical exertion increases the requirements of the body. For this reason, the heart of the elite sportsperson is usually **bigger than usual** and when at rest, it works slower than usual. In a competition, the moderate increase in the frequency of the heartbeats manages to cover all the physical requirements.

THE CARDIAC CYCLE

With each heartbeat, the four chambers in the heart dilate and contract in a **synchronized** way, allowing the blood to move from each atrium to the ventricle next to it and from there to the corresponding artery, in a cycle that goes on endlessly. The phase of cardiac **dilation** is called **diastole**, whereas the phase of cardiac **contraction** is called **systole**. On the right side, the atrium dilates and fills with the blood from the **venae cavae**. It then contracts to pump its contents into the ventricle, and finally the ventricle contracts to push the contents into the **pulmonary arteries**. On the left side, the atrium dilates and fills with blood from the **pulmonary veins**. It then contracts to pump its contents into the ventricle, which fills with blood, and finally contracts to push its contents into the **aorta**.

 The heart beats endlessly since before birth until death. Throughout a life of average length it can contract and dilate without stopping some 2500 million times.

PHASES OF THE CARDIAC CYCLE

DIASTOLE

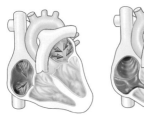

Atria relax and fill with blood from the veins

The atrioventricular valves open, allowing the passage of blood to the ventricles

ATRIAL SYSTOLE

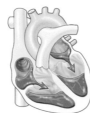

Atria contract and push their content to the ventricles

VENTRICULAR SYSTOLE

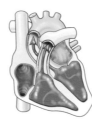

The atrioventricular valves close, and the ventricles contract to push their content to the arteries

HEART VALVES

Inside the heart, blood has a **unidirectional circulation**, which means it moves in only one direction, an essential requirement for the correct performance of the organ. This is guaranteed by a **valve** system that allows the passage of blood from one area to the other and prevents its backflow. In between each atrium and ventricle, there is an atrioventricular valve. On the right side, we find the **tricuspid valve**, so called for its shape of three small tongues. On the left side is the **mitral valve**, named for its resemblance to the miter some church dignitaries wear. In between each ventricle and the artery to which its contents are pumped, there is a **semilunar valve**; on the right side is the **pulmonary valve**, and on the left side, the **aortic valve**.

THE WORK OF THE CARDIAC VALVES

Diastole

The aortic valve is closed and prevents the backflow of blood into the right ventricle

The pulmonary valve is closed and prevents the backflow of blood into the right ventricle

The tricuspid valve opens and allows the passage of blood from the right atrium to the right ventricle

The mitral valve opens, allowing the passage of blood from the left atrium into the left ventricle

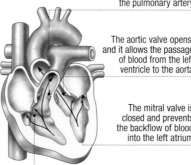

Systole

The pulmonary valve opens, allowing the passage of blood from the right ventricle to the pulmonary artery

The aortic valve opens, and it allows the passage of blood from the left ventricle to the aorta

The mitral valve is closed and prevents the backflow of blood into the left atrium

The tricuspid valve is closed and prevents the backflow of blood to the right atrium

DOUBLE CIRCUITS

Although it is a closed circuit, the circulatory system has two circuits that work in a parallel way and at the same time. The **minor circuit** is called **pulmonary circulation**. The right ventricle of the heart pumps the blood that has circulated all over the body, low in oxygen and full of carbon dioxide, to the pulmonary arteries. There it is oxygenated and once purified, it returns through the pulmonary veins to the left atrium. The **major circuit** is called **general** or **systemic circulation**. The left ventricle of the heart pushes the oxygenated blood high in nutrients to the aortic artery and its branches distributing it to all tissues. After the exchange produced in the capillaries, blood, low in oxygen and full of waste products, returns through the cavae venae.

TWO CIRCUITS OF CIRCULATION

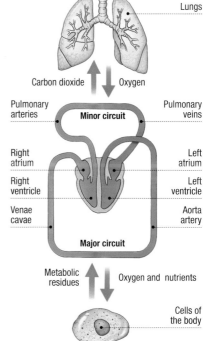

Lungs

Carbon dioxide / Oxygen

Pulmonary arteries — Minor circuit — Pulmonary veins

Right atrium — Left atrium

Right ventricle — Left ventricle

Venae cavae — Aorta artery

Major circuit

Metabolic residues / Oxygen and nutrients

Cells of the body

CARDIAC AUTOMATISM

Heartbeats depend on **electric stimuli** that cause the contraction of fibers that form the **cardiac muscle** and that cause a consecutive and synchronized contraction of the organ's chambers. Those stimuli are generated in a rhythmic way in specific areas of the heart and spread in a sequence along the organ through specialized muscular fibers that constitute the **system of electric conduction**. Thus, although cardiac activity can be influenced by stimuli from the nervous system that may accelerate or slow down the rate of its beats, the heart is an organ **autonomous in function**.

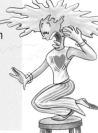

Heart rate refers to the number of heartbeats that occur in one minute, some 70 or 80 times in an adult when at rest, a little higher in children and a little lower in elderly people. However, the heart rate can increase when making a physical effort and in stressful situations.

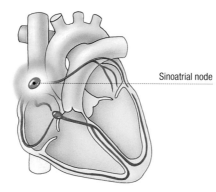

1
Stimuli are generated in the sinoatrial node, located in the right atrium

Sinoatrial node

Internodal tracts

2
From there, they spread through internodal pathways in the right and left atria, causing a contraction in both chambers

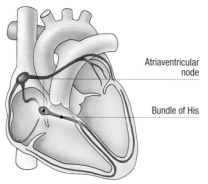

3
Then they get to the atrioventricular node, located by the orifice that connects the atrium and ventricle on the right and continue traveling through the bundle of His, which heads for to the interventricular septum

Atriaventricular node

Bundle of His

Left and right branches

Purkinje's network

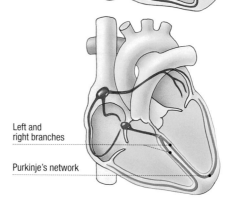

4
The stimuli spread through the right and left bundle branches and finally go to the Purkinje fibers, a complex network of ramifications that expand along the walls of the two ventricles, causing the contraction of these chambers

HEART INNERVATION

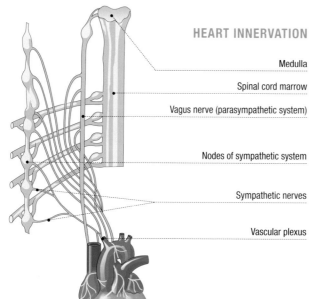

Medulla

Spinal cord marrow

Vagus nerve (parasympathetic system)

Nodes of sympathetic system

Sympathetic nerves

Vascular plexus

NERVOUS CONTROL OF THE HEART

Although the heart works autonomously, it is innervated by the **autonomic nervous system**, the part of the central nervous system that controls the activity of the internal organs **involuntarily**. Fibers from both parts of the autonomic nervous system (**sympathetic system** and **parasympathetic system**) connect to the heart. The stimuli provided by these areas have opposite effects. The sympathetic system activates when there is a physical effort or when there is an intense emotion, causing an increase in the heart rate, while the parasympathetic system, which predominates when we are relaxed and at rest, results in a slowing down of the heartbeat.

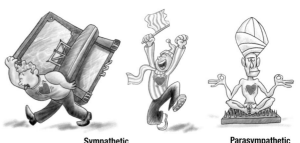

Sympathetic nervous system

Parasympathetic nervous system

Introduction

A Perfect Machine

Skin

Digestive System

Nutrition

Respiratory System

Circulatory System and Blood

Nervous System

Musculoskeletal System

Urinary System

Endocrine System

Immune System

The Senses

Genetics

Reproductive System

Human Development

Index

BLOOD PRESSURE

The blood pressure corresponds to the **pressure** that blood exerts against the walls of the arteries when pumped by the heart with each heartbeat. Pressure is **needed** to **ensure circulation**, because blood must **overcome the resistance** associated with the progressive decrease in diameter of the arterial vessels. With each contraction, the left ventricle propels some blood to the aorta, whose ramifications become thinner and thinner. The blood is distributed throughout the body. The aorta and the main arteries are elastic, so at first they distend and then they return to their previous diameter. The blood is propelled to the minor vessels and a practically continuous flow is established in the capillaries. There are two factors that determine the blood pressure: **heart output**, which corresponds to the amount of blood expelled by the heart in each minute, and **peripheral vascular resistance**, which corresponds to the opposition of the small arteries, more or less contracted or relaxed.

IS THE HEART THE HOUSE OF LOVE?

Traditionally, it is thought that the heart hosts our feelings, that it is where love resides. However, it is only a fantasy, romantic, but unreal. Maybe the idea was conceived upon realization that when we feel moved, the heart beats faster, but it is just an automatic response to the stimuli from the nervous system. Moreover, it can be stated that the heart is an insensitive organ, because it lacks nerve endings sensitive to either touch or temperature. However, it has receptors that activate and cause pain when certain metabolic products collect because of poor blood irrigation.

SYSTOLIC AND DIASTOLIC BLOOD PRESSURE

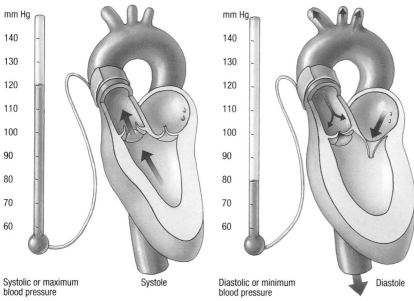

Systolic or maximum blood pressure — Systole

Diastolic or minimum blood pressure — Diastole

The blood pressure is the parameter indicating the level of health of the circulatory system.

BLOOD PRESSURE (BP) NORMAL RANGES

Age	Systolic BP	Diastolic BP
1–3 months	80	55
4–12	90	65
1–4 years old	110	70
5–10 years old	110	70
11–15 yrs old	110	70
16–20 yrs old	120	80
21–30 yrs old	120	80
31–40 yrs old	120	80
41–50 yrs old	120	80
51–60 yrs old	120	80
61–70 yrs old	120	80
+ 70 years old	120	80

VARIATIONS IN BLOOD PRESSURE

The blood pressure is not uniform; it presents certain oscillations in the course of a heartbeat. For that reason, two parameters are always taken into consideration when referring to its value: maximum and minimum blood pressure expressed in **mercury millimeters** (mm Hg). **Maximum** or **systolic blood pressure** corresponds to systole, that is, the phase in which the left ventricle pumps its contents into the aorta whose internal pressure increases abruptly. **Minimum** or **diastolic blood pressure** corresponds to diastole, the phase in which the left ventricle dilates to fill up and therefore does not discharge blood into the aorta. It is worth mentioning that the blood pressure presents several variations throughout the day and that its values increase progressively with age. Under normal conditions, they stay within certain ranges.

ARTERIAL CIRCULATION

MECHANISM OF ARTERIAL CIRCULATION

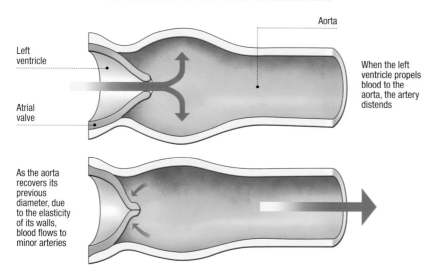

Left ventricle

Atrial valve

Aorta

When the left ventricle propels blood to the aorta, the artery distends

As the aorta recovers its previous diameter, due to the elasticity of its walls, blood flows to minor arteries

Major arteries, such as the aorta and its main branches, have **elastic walls** that allow them to **expand** when the heart vigorously expels a large amount of blood with each heartbeat, and to go back to their previous diameter later. They propel the blood to the rest of the arterial tree, formed by thinner and thinner vessels that are less elastic. This mechanism transforms an intermittent gush of blood into a **continuous flow**. Minor arteries, however, have a larger proportion of muscular fibers in their walls, and, under the influence of the nervous system, they can be more contracted or relaxed. This mechanism allows the **distribution** of blood throughout the body, so that the areas needing a greater supply can receive it at all times as, for example, the muscles during exercise or the digestive system during digestion.

ARTERIAL PULSE

Each time the heart contracts, it **propels** blood to the aortic artery, which distributes the blood throughout the body by means of its ramifications. As the blood flow moves through these vessels with elastic walls, during its passage it also spreads a **pulse wave** that corresponds to the contraction of the left ventricle. So, when touching the pulsation of **superficial arteries**, valuable information is obtained about the rhythm and the rate of the heart. To take the pulse, you just need to place the tips of the fingers on top of a medium size artery to detect its pulsations. Indeed, you can take your own pulse without much difficulty. Generally, you take the pulse of the **radial artery** on its path by the edge of the inside face of the wrist, by the thumb. It is also easy to detect the pulsation of the **carotid arteries** in the neck, on the sides of the trachea, and also the **femoral arteries** in the groin.

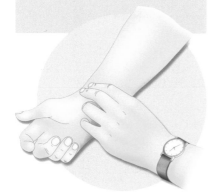

VENOUS CIRCULATION

Veins are responsible for **return circulation**. They are in charge of carrying blood to the heart from every point of the body. In the veins located in the upper area of the body, this circulation is possible simply because the venous walls are able to dilate and the existent pressure inside is lower than that in the right atrium, which has an "aspiration" effect. The veins located in the lower area of the body are different, especially when you are on your feet, because the blood moves to the heart **against gravity**. These vessels also have a system of **internal valves** that only allow the blood to move in one direction, toward the heart, preventing it from backing up. Besides, there is a **muscular pump** in the lower extremities, because the veins run in between the muscles and when these muscles contract they provide the necessary impulse for venous circulation.

MECHANISM OF VENOUS CIRCULATION IN LOWER PART OF BODY

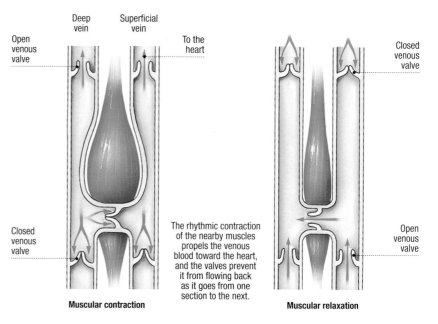

Deep vein

Superficial vein

Open venous valve

To the heart

Closed venous valve

Closed venous valve

Open venous valve

The rhythmic contraction of the nearby muscles propels the venous blood toward the heart, and the valves prevent it from flowing back as it goes from one section to the next.

Muscular contraction

Muscular relaxation

CAPILLARY CIRCULATION

The capillaries are the **last branches** of peripheral arteries. They are the smallest vessels, even thinner than a hair, which is where their name comes from. Their walls formed by one layer of cells are so thin that they allow exchanges between the blood circulating inside them and their surrounding area. The blood that reaches the capillaries in a continuous flow is full of oxygen and nutrients. These elements pass through the capillary walls and are caught by cells in nearby tissues. At the same time, carbon dioxide and other metabolic residues pass from the tissues into the blood, which slowly becomes venous blood. When the capillaries meet, veins begin to form, which will carry the impure blood to the heart.

LYMPHATIC SYSTEM

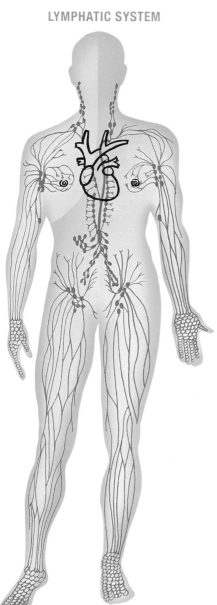

Introduction

A Perfect Machine

Skin

Digestive System

Nutrition

Respiratory System

Circulatory System and Blood

Nervous System

Musculoskeletal System

Urinary System

Endocrine System

Immune System

The Senses

Genetics

Reproductive System

Human Development

Index

EXCHANGES IN CAPILLARY CIRCULATION

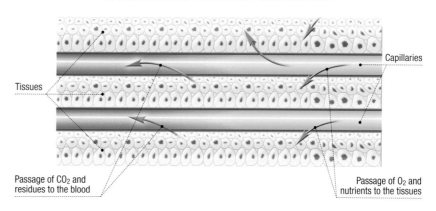

Tissues

Capillaries

Passage of CO_2 and residues to the blood

Passage of O_2 and nutrients to the tissues

LYMPHATIC SYSTEM

The lymphatic system is part of the circulatory system, and it is in charge of **draining** or **collecting** surplus fluid in the intercellular spaces of several tissues. It is also part of the **immune system**. It is made up of a complex **network of ducts**, which are very thin. These ducts drain some of the fluid leaking from the capillaries and direct it back into the bloodstream, pick up the fats absorbed in the digestive system, and collect proteins, germs, and small particles present in tissues. **Lymph capillaries** come together to form **lymph vessels**, larger in diameter, that go to the heart. Along their path, there are **nodes** that filter the fluid they transport—**lymph**. Finally, all lymph vessels come together at two main ducts that connect to veins close to the superior vena cava.

CIRCULATION IN THE LYMPH VESSELS

Lymph vessels do not have a central pump equivalent to the heart. Their performance depends especially on their **compression** caused by adjacent muscles. A regular decrease in pressure that occurs inside the thoracic cage during inhalation makes it easy for the lymph to go up from the legs to the trunk of the body. Inside the lymph vessels, there is a **valve system** that ensures lymph circulation in just one direction and prevents its backflow.

RELATIONSHIP BETWEEN LYMPH CIRCULATION AND BLOOD CIRCULATION

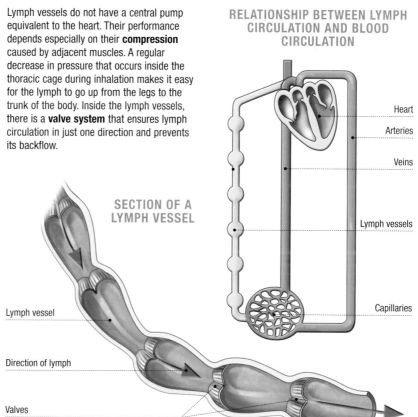

Heart

Arteries

Veins

Lymph vessels

Capillaries

SECTION OF A LYMPH VESSEL

Lymph vessel

Direction of lymph

Valves

BLOOD, A VITAL FLUID

Blood is a **reddish** viscous **fluid** that is pumped by the heart. It travels throughout the whole body constantly, via the circulatory system. It has, among other functions, that of **transporting many elements** to tissue cells to support their activity and also transporting waste products to the organs in charge of their elimination.

BLOOD COMPOSITION

BLOOD COMPONENTS

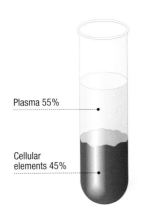

Plasma 55%

Cellular elements 45%

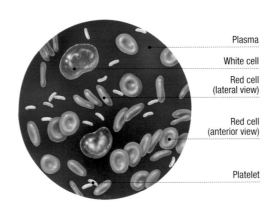

Plasma
White cell
Red cell (lateral view)
Red cell (anterior view)
Platelet

In an adult, there are approximately **5 liters** of blood, made up of different components. Approximately 55% of the blood corresponds to **plasma**, a fluid that carries many dissolved substances. In the plasma, thousands of millions of various **cellular elements** float; they constitute the other 45% of the blood. There are three types of blood cells, each one with a different function. **Red cells** are responsible for transporting oxygen and carbon dioxide. There are different varieties of **white cells**, but their role is to take part in the defense of the body against infections. **Platelets** take part in the coagulation process, which stops bleeding.

BLOOD CELLS

Red cells	4.5–5 million/mm³
White cells	4,000–10,000/mm³
• Neutrophils	45–75%
• Eosinophils	1–3%
• Basophils	0.5–1%
• Monocytes	3–7%
• Lymphocytes	25–30%
• Platelets	150,000-300,000/mm³

Red cells are also known as **erythrocytes**; white cells are also called **leukocytes**, and platelets are also called **thrombocytes**.

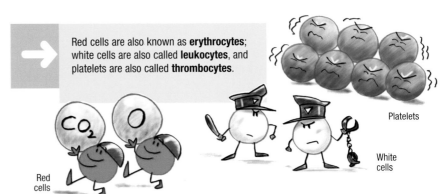

Platelets

White cells

Red cells

THE FUNCTION OF BLOOD

Blood has different functions, but above all, it acts as a **vehicle** for several materials. It transports them inside the body; on the one hand, it delivers to all tissues the oxygen absorbed in the lungs, the nutrients acquired by the digestive system, the hormones produced by endocrine glands, and multiple elements necessary for the healthy performance of the cells. On the other hand, it carries the residues of cellular metabolism, whose buildup would be toxic, to the organs in charge of their elimination or neutralization, such as kidneys and lungs. Blood also takes part in **thermoregulation** of the body, because it acts as a heating system distributing heat and keeping the right temperature for the proper performance of tissues. Finally, it also helps with the **defense system** that protects against infections.

BLOOD PLASMA

Plasma is a **yellowish fluid** mainly made up of water (90%) that transports blood cells and elements, such as **nutrients**, **residues** of metabolism, **vitamins**, **hormones**, and several products of diverse biological actions. Nutrients, such as sugars, fats, and amino acids; residues of metabolism, such as urea; and some materials travel freely in the plasma. But many are insoluble and form complexes with proteins that secure them to release them in the corresponding place. As a matter of fact, among the main components of plasma, there are several **proteins**, the main ones being **albumins**.

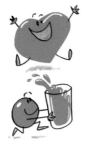

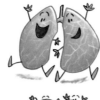

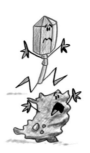

The three types of blood cells and their functions.

BLOOD FORMATION

Blood cell formation is a continuous process, called **hematopoiesis**, taking place mainly in the **bone marrow**, which is inside of some bones. In a lesser degree, it also takes place in the immune system organs, such as the spleen and lymph nodes. There are some **pluripotent stem cells** (precursor cells of all blood cells) in the bone marrow. They are able to reproduce and to differentiate to create monopotent stem cells, prepared for a specific type of blood cell. From their beginning, blood elements go through a **maturation process**, receiving different names as they advance in stages, finally becoming red cells, white cells, or platelets that will go into the blood stream. Because blood cells have a limited life, each day an amount is produced to replenish the losses. That represents some astronomical figures: 100,000 to 200,000 million red cells, approximately 30,000 million white cells, and between 70,000 and 150,000 million platelets.

If all red cells of an adult were placed in a line, one after the other, it would be possible to form a chain that would go around the Earth more than five times.

HEMATOPOIESIS

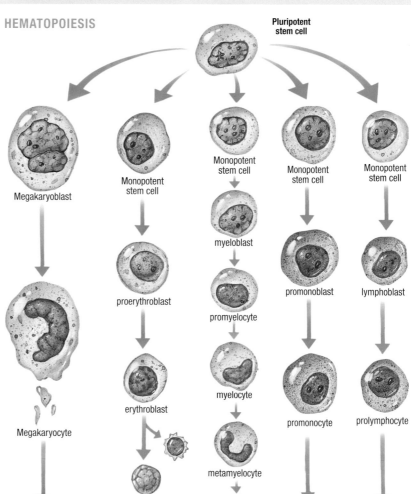

Pluripotent stem cell

Megakaryoblast

Monopotent stem cell

Monopotent stem cell

Monopotent stem cell

Monopotent stem cell

myeloblast

proerythroblast

promyelocyte

promonoblast

lymphoblast

erythroblast

myelocyte

Megakaryocyte

promonocyte

prolymphocyte

metamyelocyte

reticulocyte

band cells

monocyte

lymphocyte

Platelet

red cell

granulocyte

THE LIFE OF RED CELLS

Red cells are **incomplete cells**, because they lack a nucleus and that means that after some time of circulating throughout the body they lose vitality and are destroyed. They are formed in the bone marrow from pluripotent cells in a process called **erythropoiesis** that lasts between 5 and eight days. From the bone marrow they go to the blood to play their role. On average, they remain in perfect condition to perform their function for about three months. After that period, once they get old, red cells are destroyed when passing through the **spleen**.

DONATE BLOOD, DONATE LIFE

Blood banks need large amounts of blood in order to respond to multiple situations (accidents, surgeries, transplants, etc.). To qualify as a donor and help save lives, a person has to be between 18 and 65 years old, weigh over 80 pounds, and be in good health.

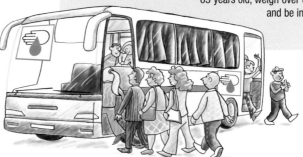

Introduction

A Perfect Machine

Skin

Digestive System

Nutrition

Respiratory System

Circulatory System and Blood

Nervous System

Musculoskeletal System

Urinary System

Endocrine System

Immune System

The Senses

Genetics

Reproductive System

Human Development

Index

FUNCTION OF RED CELLS

Red cells have a **vital function**: they are in charge of **transporting oxygen** from the lungs to the tissues, where cells use it in their metabolic processes. They also transport **carbon dioxide** from the tissues to the lungs to be eliminated and to prevent its buildup. This function is carried out by a **pigment**, **hemoglobin**, which is contained in red cells, and is also responsible for giving blood its characteristic coloration. It could be said that red blood cells act simply as hemoglobin "containers," because their purpose is to travel inside the circulatory system going through the lungs and tissues repeatedly so that the pigment can transport those gases back and forth.

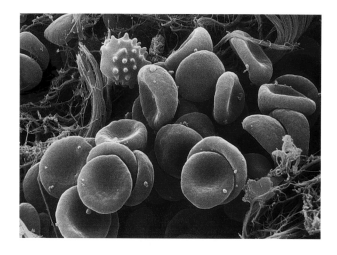

Red cells seen through a scanning microscope.

NORMAL LEVELS OF RED CELLS AND HEMOGLOBIN ACCORDING TO AGE AND GENDER

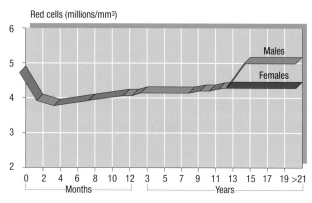

Red cells (millions/mm³)

Males
Females

Months — Years

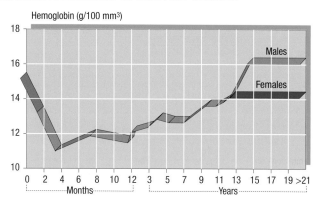

Hemoglobin (g/100 mm³)

Males
Females

Months — Years

STRUCTURE OF HEMOGLOBIN

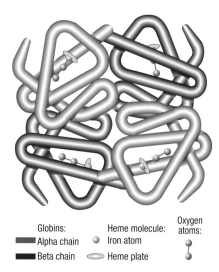

Globins:
— Alpha chain
— Beta chain

Heme molecule:
○ Iron atom
⬭ Heme plate

Oxygen atoms:

When hemoglobin is full of oxygen, it has a bright red color, characteristic of arterial blood. But when it is full of carbon dioxide it has a bluer color characteristic of venous blood.

HEMOGLOBIN

Hemoglobin is made up of two essential elements from which its name derives: one compound called **heme group** and some proteins of a **globin** type. Each hemoglobin molecule has four heme groups combined in four chains of globins. The heme group has one iron atom that is capable of binding oxygen to transport it in the blood. When it becomes exposed to a high concentration of oxygen, as when it passes through the lungs, each hemoglobin molecule can affix four molecules of oxygen, which join the corresponding iron atoms; thus oxyhemoglobin occurs, having a bright red color. When the concentration of oxygen decreases and carbon dioxide concentration increases, hemoglobin releases oxygen to give it to the tissues. At the same time, hemoglobin incorporates a molecule of carbon dioxide to transport it to the lungs, becoming **carboxyhemoglobin**, which has a bluish color. Hemoglobin passes the carbon dioxide to the lungs to be eliminated through breathing and one more time it incorporates oxygen, beginning anew the continuous cycle that ensures the gas exchange between the body and the outside.

FUNCTION OF HEMOGLOBIN

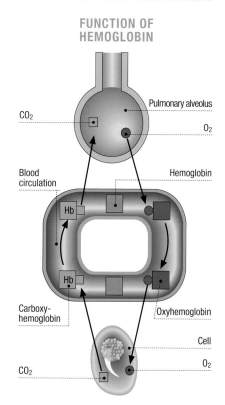

CO_2
Pulmonary alveolus
O_2

Blood circulation
Hemoglobin

Hb
Hb

Carboxy-hemoglobin
Oxyhemoglobin

Cell

CO_2
O_2

STRUCTURE OF THE SPLEEN

Outside view

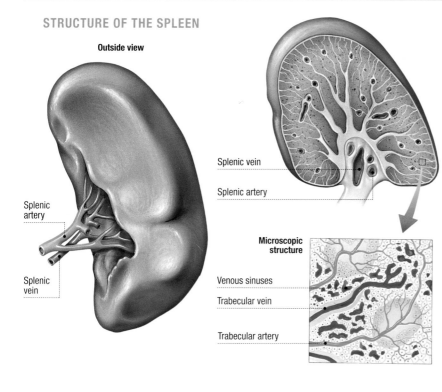

Splenic artery

Splenic vein

Splenic vein

Splenic artery

Microscopic structure

Venous sinuses

Trabecular vein

Trabecular artery

FUNCTIONS OF THE SPLEEN

The spleen is a spongy organ, which under normal conditions, is full of blood. One of its functions is to provide a **blood reservoir** that empties into the bloodstream in any emergency situation, such as when there is severe bleeding. But the main function of the spleen is to **destroy worn out red cells**. When red cells lose their vitality and their walls get deformed, they stay trapped in the spleen and are destroyed, although their components go to the blood to be recycled, especially the iron in hemoglobin.

WHITE CELLS

White cells are also called **leukocytes**. They are the least numerous blood cells and are of different types. They all have a nucleus, and some of them have a multilobed nucleus that, when seen under the microscope, appears to be more than one. There are two groups of white cells: multinuclear and mononuclear. **Multinuclear leukocytes** are also called **granulocytes**, because when they are studied under the microscope, they show granules

inside. These granules contain needed materials for their leukocyte activity. There are three different subgroups: **neutrophils**, **eosinophils**, and **basophils**. Mononuclear leukocytes are of two kinds: **monocytes**, the largest blood cells, and **lymphocytes**, which are much smaller but more numerous. These lymphocytes are classified according to their activity into **B-lymphocytes** and **T-lymphocytes**.

ANEMIA

Anemia is a very **common disorder**, characterized by a decrease in the levels of hemoglobin and a decrease in red cell concentration. Consequently anemia manifests as paleness and fatigue, because the tissues cannot receive all the oxygen needed for their proper performance. Causes of anemia can be extremely varied: some times it is **bleeding** that causes an exaggerated or repeated **loss** of red cells and the hemoglobin in them; other times, it is a **failure** in the formation of hemoglobin or red cells, either because of genetic reasons or caused by a **depletion** of needed elements, such as iron, folic acid, or vitamin B_{12}.

TYPES OF WHITE CELLS

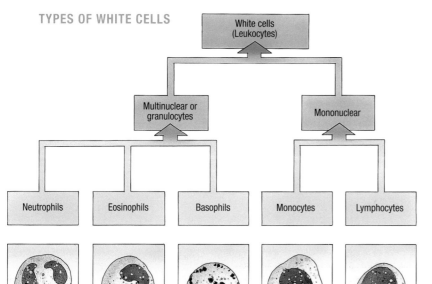

White cells (Leukocytes)

Multinuclear or granulocytes — Mononuclear

Neutrophils | Eosinophils | Basophils | Monocytes | Lymphocytes

All white cells take part in the **immune system** and although some stay in the blood during a large part of their active life, others leave the circulatory system to penetrate different organic tissues and defend against foreign objects.

51

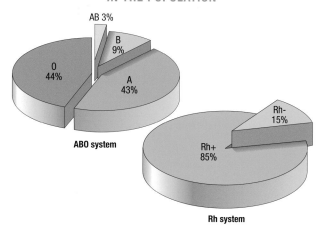

FREQUENCY OF BLOOD TYPES IN THE POPULATION

AB 3%

B 9%

O 44%

A 43%

ABO system

Rh- 15%

Rh+ 85%

Rh system

BLOOD TYPES

In humans, blood is classified in different groups, depending on the presence or the absence of certain antigens on the surface of red cells. Their existence is determined **genetically** and is subjected to hereditary laws. This classification determines the degree of **blood compatibility**, that is, the possibility of using blood from one individual to give transfusions to another one without resulting problems. When you give blood from one person with a particular blood type, to another person with a different blood type, the donor's red cells introduced in the recipient's bloodstream may be attacked and destroyed by the antibodies present in the plasma. That would cause an **incompatibility reaction**, which could be slight and temporary, but, in other cases, it could be so severe that it could be fatal. Several antigens have been identified on the surface of the red cells, but the most important ones that are taken into consideration when giving blood are the ones corresponding to ABO system and Rh factor.

ABO SYSTEM

The ABO system is based on the existence of two antigens in the surface of red cells, named A and B. Depending on the presence or the absence of one or both antigens, four different blood types can be distinguished. In **type A blood**, only the A antigen is present. In **type B blood**, only the B antigen is present. In **type AB blood**, both antigens are present, and, in the **O group**, neither is present. At the same time, the absence of a particular antigen on the surface of the red cells is associated with the presence in the plasma of **specific antibodies** against that antigen responsible for incompatibility reactions. Thus, in type A blood there are **anti-B antibodies** and in type B blood, there are **anti-A antibodies**. In type O blood, there are anti-A and anti-B antigens; however blood type AB has neither one.

THE ABO BLOOD TYPE SYSTEM

BLOOD TYPE	SURFACE ANTIGEN	ANTIBODY
A	A	anti-B
B	B	anti-A
AB	A B	
O		anti-A anti-B

BLOOD COMPATIBILITY

If someone from group A were to have a type B **blood transfusion**, the anti-B antibodies present in the plasma of the recipient would react against the donor's red cells containing B antigen and they would destroy them. The same would happen if type A blood were used to transfuse a type B blood individual, because the anti-A antibodies in the plasma would destroy the red cells of the blood received. However, if a type AB person were given a different type blood, there would be hardly any problems, because there are no anti-A or anti-B antigens present and therefore the red cells would not be attacked. A person with a type AB blood is considered a "**universal recipient**." However, an individual with a type O blood cannot be given blood from any other blood type, because the plasma contains antibodies that would destroy the red cells given. Type O red cells do not have any surface antigen, so they can be given to people from other groups without any risks: people with type O blood type are considered "**universal donors.**"

TRANSFUSION COMPATIBILITY OF THE ABO SYSTEM

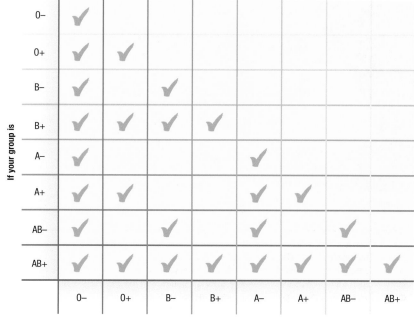

If your group is	0–	0+	B–	B+	A–	A+	AB–	AB+
0–	✓							
0+	✓	✓						
B–	✓		✓					
B+	✓	✓	✓	✓				
A–	✓				✓			
A+	✓	✓			✓	✓		
AB–	✓		✓		✓		✓	
AB+	✓	✓	✓	✓	✓	✓	✓	✓

you can be given

BLOOD, A VITAL FLUID

Introduction

A Perfect Machine

Skin

Digestive System

Nutrition

Respiratory System

Circulatory System and Blood

Nervous System

Musculoskeletal System

Urinary System

Endocrine System

Immune System

The Senses

Genetics

Reproductive System

Human Development

Index

Rh FACTOR

Rh factor is an antigen on the surface of red cells present in approximately 85% of people considered **Rh positive** (Rh+). Rh factor is absent in the rest, who are considered **Rh negative** (Rh–). If blood from a person with Rh+ is given to an individual with Rh–, the recipient generates anti-Rh antibodies that destroy the transfused red cells. Therefore, blood from an individual with Rh– can be given to people with Rh+ but not the other way around.

In cases of blood incompatibility between mother and child (mother Rh negative and baby Rh positive) anti-Rh immunoglobulin must be administered to the pregnant woman to prevent hemolytic disease of newborn (HDN).

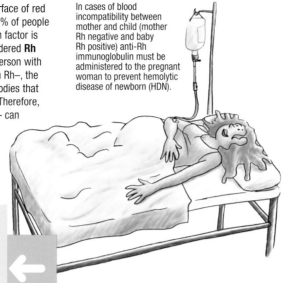

Rh factor is called so because it is also present in a type of monkey called Macacus rhesus, where it was first identified.

COMPATIBILITY IN BLOOD TRANSFUSION Rh FACTOR

		Donor	
	Rh Factor	Rh+	Rh–
Recipient	Rh+	compatible	compatible
	Rh–	incompatible	compatible

Blood clot seen under the microscope

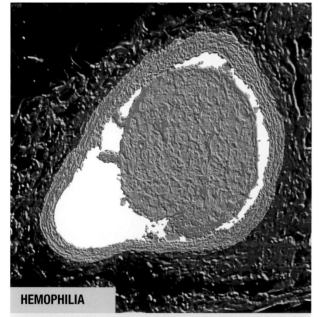

HEMOPHILIA

Hemophilia is an alteration of blood clotting caused by a genetic defect. It causes an absence or a decrease of some of the clotting factors. The degree of this alteration results in more or less serious consequences for the person who suffers it. Hemophilia is transmitted from parents to children, making it a hereditary disease (anomaly), linked to gender, X-chromosome. It is suffered almost exclusively by males and is transmitted by females.

FUNCTION OF PLATELETS: COAGULATION

Platelets are the smallest corpuscles in the blood. They participate actively in the **coagulation** (clotting) **mechanism** whose purpose is to stop **bleeding** caused by wounds in blood vessels and to prevent **blood loss**. Coagulation is a very complex process, where not only the platelets take part but also other materials present in plasma called **coagulation factors** are involved. When a vessel tears, the platelets clump upon each other in the hole and release one of those clotting factors, which activates the others. The final objective of those reactions is to take a material dissolved in the plasma, **fibrinogen**, and turn it into a solid material, **fibrin**. This material adheres to the platelets and other blood elements, forming a solid clot that seals the opening.

CLOTTING MECHANISM

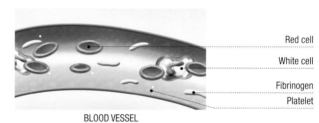

Red cell

White cell

Fibrinogen

Platelet

BLOOD VESSEL

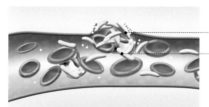

The platelets collect in the wound

THE WOUND OCCURS

Fibrin

Fibrinogen

FIBRINOGEN TURNS INTO FIBRIN

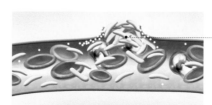

Fibrin network

A CLOT FORMS

THE NERVOUS SYSTEM

The nervous system **regulates** all the works of the body; it is responsible for both our **voluntary conscious acts** and the automatic nonconscious activity of the many body organs. It is in charge of the **relationship** with the environment and it is the seat of **intellectual activity**. It controls our lives completely.

COMPONENTS OF THE NERVOUS SYSTEM

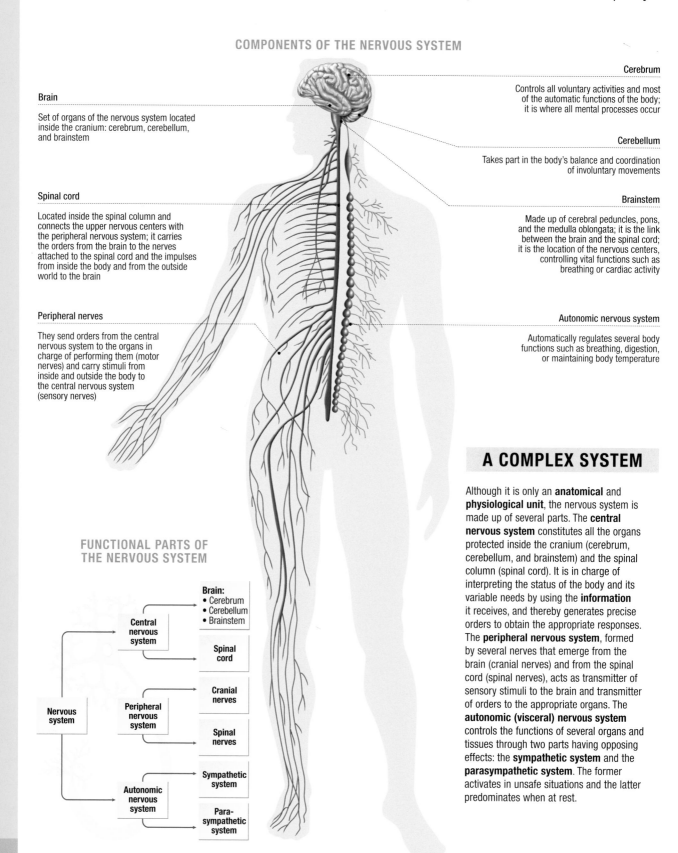

Brain

Set of organs of the nervous system located inside the cranium: cerebrum, cerebellum, and brainstem

Spinal cord

Located inside the spinal column and connects the upper nervous centers with the peripheral nervous system; it carries the orders from the brain to the nerves attached to the spinal cord and the impulses from inside the body and from the outside world to the brain

Peripheral nerves

They send orders from the central nervous system to the organs in charge of performing them (motor nerves) and carry stimuli from inside and outside the body to the central nervous system (sensory nerves)

Cerebrum

Controls all voluntary activities and most of the automatic functions of the body; it is where all mental processes occur

Cerebellum

Takes part in the body's balance and coordination of involuntary movements

Brainstem

Made up of cerebral peduncles, pons, and the medulla oblongata; it is the link between the brain and the spinal cord; it is the location of the nervous centers, controlling vital functions such as breathing or cardiac activity

Autonomic nervous system

Automatically regulates several body functions such as breathing, digestion, or maintaining body temperature

FUNCTIONAL PARTS OF THE NERVOUS SYSTEM

Nervous system

- **Central nervous system**
  - **Brain:**
    - Cerebrum
    - Cerebellum
    - Brainstem
  - **Spinal cord**
- **Peripheral nervous system**
  - **Cranial nerves**
  - **Spinal nerves**
- **Autonomic nervous system**
  - **Sympathetic system**
  - **Para-sympathetic system**

A COMPLEX SYSTEM

Although it is only an **anatomical** and **physiological unit**, the nervous system is made up of several parts. The **central nervous system** constitutes all the organs protected inside the cranium (cerebrum, cerebellum, and brainstem) and the spinal column (spinal cord). It is in charge of interpreting the status of the body and its variable needs by using the **information** it receives, and thereby generates precise orders to obtain the appropriate responses. The **peripheral nervous system**, formed by several nerves that emerge from the brain (cranial nerves) and from the spinal cord (spinal nerves), acts as transmitter of sensory stimuli to the brain and transmitter of orders to the appropriate organs. The **autonomic (visceral) nervous system** controls the functions of several organs and tissues through two parts having opposing effects: the **sympathetic system** and the **parasympathetic system**. The former activates in unsafe situations and the latter predominates when at rest.

Introduction

A Perfect
Machine

Skin

Digestive
System

Nutrition

Respiratory
System

Circulatory
System and
Blood

**Nervous
System**

Musculoskeletal
System

Urinary
System

Endocrine
System

Immune
System

The Senses

Genetics

Reproductive
System

Human
Development

Index

STRUCTURE OF A NEURON

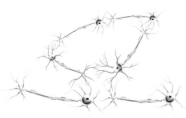

Cell
body

Nucleus

Dendrites

Myelin sheath

Axon

Axonal tree (terminal synapses)

RELATIONSHIP OF NEURONS

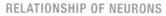

HOW THE NERVOUS IMPULSE IS GENERATED

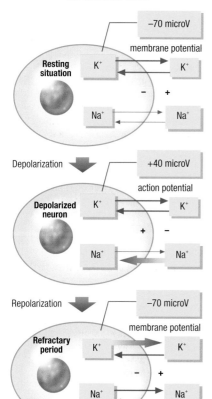

−70 microV

membrane potential

Resting situation

K⁺   K⁺

−   +

Na⁺   Na⁺

Depolarization

+40 microV

action potential

Depolarized neuron

K⁺   K⁺

+   −

Na⁺   Na⁺

Repolarization

−70 microV

membrane potential

Refractary period

K⁺   K⁺

−   +

Na⁺   Na⁺

NERVE TISSUE

All components of the nervous system, from the brain to the simplest nerve, are made up of specialized cells: **neurons**. They constitute a **complex network** and are closely related to one another, because the system's functioning depends on its interconnections. Nerve cells vary in appearance and size, but they all have a **cell body** containing extensions in charge of receiving and transmitting nervous impulses from and to other neurons. **Dendrites** are short branches that receive the stimuli from other nerve cells. The **axon** is an extension of variable length that ends in tiny branches and is responsible for transmitting impulses to other nerve cells.

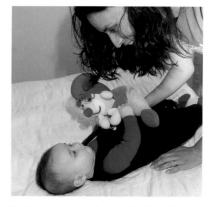

The human nervous system consists of over 100 billion neurons.

Neurons are the only cells in the body that do not replicate during the course of one's life.

NERVE IMPULSE

Neurons communicate with each other by using signals transmitted by a complex physicochemical mechanism: nervous impulses. Some biochemical changes occur in the neuron in the presence of certain stimuli. These chemical changes trigger an electric signal that goes through the cell along the axon and to the axon's end where the communication with adjacent neurons occurs. In all neurons, there is always a difference in the electric charge between the inside and the outside of the cellular membrane. At rest, there is a positive electric charge outside with respect to the one inside. This difference is called **membrane potential**, which is maintained by a "sodium pump" outside the cell that causes the sodium ions to leave the cell. If a stimulus causes a sudden increase of permeability in the membrane, there is an increase in the positive charge inside so the membrane is said to **depolarize**. If a stimulus reaches a certain degree an **action potential** is triggered, so that the current spreads all over the cell, to the end of the axon. To return to its resting state, a "potassium pump" acts, causing the potassium ions to leave. During this process, called **repolarization**, there is a **refractory period** in which a neuron is not able to generate or receive a new impulse: only after that time period passes can a new action potential occur.

SPREAD OF NERVOUS IMPULSE

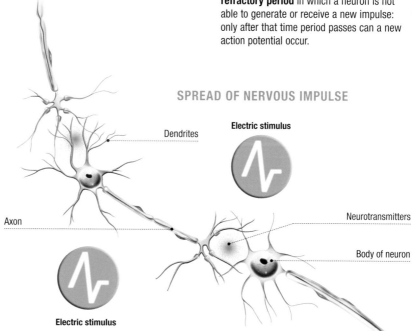

Dendrites

Electric stimulus

Axon

Electric stimulus

Neurotransmitters

Body of neuron

TRANSMISSION OF NERVE IMPULSE

SYNAPSE

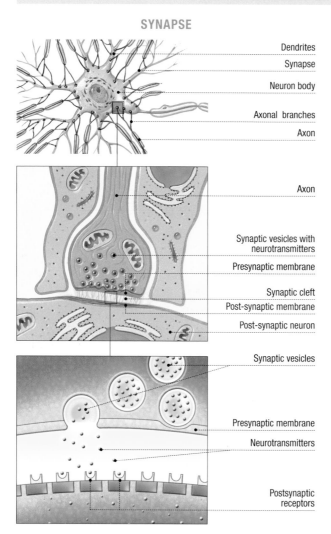

Dendrites
Synapse
Neuron body
Axonal branches
Axon

Axon

Synaptic vesicles with neurotransmitters
Presynaptic membrane
Synaptic cleft
Post-synaptic membrane
Post-synaptic neuron

Synaptic vesicles

Presynaptic membrane
Neurotransmitters

Postsynaptic receptors

Nerve impulses are not transmitted to adjacent neurons through direct contact but through a special connection called a **synapse**. Axonal branches end very close to adjacent neurons, but a narrow space called a **synaptic fissure** separates them. Nervous impulses go through that space by means of a chemical called a **neurotransmitter**. Each neuron makes a specific neurotransmitter, which is stored in the **synaptic vesicles** located in the axonal branches. When an electric impulse arrives to the extreme of the axon, these vesicles release their content into the synaptic fissure. When going through this space, the neurotransmitter combines with receptors present on the surface of adjacent neurons and this generates chemical changes in the membrane, whose effect depends on the type of neurotransmitter: it can trigger an electric potential (excitatory synapse), or, quite the opposite, it can reduce its excitability (inhibiting synapse). If the stimuli trigger an action potential, an electric signal will be generated that will go through the cell to the end of the axon and will cause the release of its neurotransmitter in the corresponding synapse, thus spreading the information.

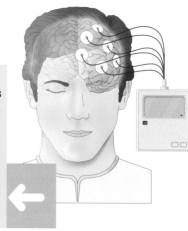

Electric currents that constitute nerve impulses are very weak, but they can still be detected on the surface of the body: for example you can record the brain activity by doing an ECG.

Each neuron establishes synapses with several, sometimes thousands, of nearby neurons. Their activity depends on the sum of all the excitatory and inhibiting stimuli that are being received all the time.

GRAY MATTER, WHITE MATTER

In most neurons, the axon is covered with a **wrapping** made up of a series of concentric layers of a **fatty whitish substance** called the **myelin sheath**, which is produced by specialized cells: **oligodendrocytes or Schwann cells**. This myelin sheath has insulating properties and is very important for the appropriate transmission of nerve impulses. In the organs of the central nervous system, there are areas made up of neuron bodies, whereas others have bundles of nerve fibers corresponding to the cellular extensions, the axons. In the first case, we speak of "**gray matter**," because this is the predominant color in neuron bodies. However, the bundles of nerve fibers, each surrounded by a whitish myelin sheath, constitute the so-called **white matter**.

MYELIN SHEATH

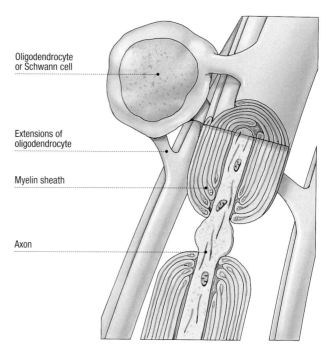

Oligodendrocyte or Schwann cell

Extensions of oligodendrocyte

Myelin sheath

Axon

THE CENTRAL NERVOUS SYSTEM: A HUGE COMPUTER

There are some who compare the central nervous system with a **powerful computer**. Actually the simile is not accurate, because it is much more complex than the most complex computer. It is true that it **processes** and elaborates endless information from different channels just like a computer does. It has a **central unit** that deals with all that information; it stores some of it and sends appropriate answers to the different organs according to each situation. The brain corresponds to the central unit, and it sends and receives data through the brainstem and two intermediate stations: the cerebellum and the spinal cord. The peripheral nerves are something like the wires in charge of sending messages to and from the appropriate organs.

MOTOR AND SENSORY AREAS

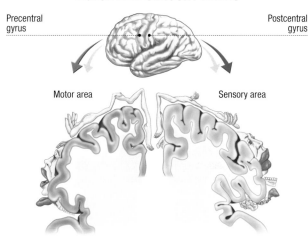

Precentral gyrus

Postcentral gyrus

Motor area

Sensory area

In the motor and sensory areas of the cerebral cortex, there is a correlation between each section and the parts of the body that require a more precise motor control or from which more sensory stimuli are received.

CEREBRAL AREAS

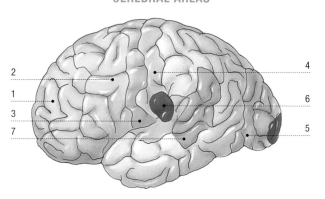

1. Frontal area: superior mental functions
2. Premotor area: control of head and eye movements
3. Motor area: control of voluntary movements
4. Sensory area: perception and interpretation of body sensations
5. Visual area
6. Auditory area
7. Language area

FUNCTIONS OF BRAIN

The brain controls all the basic functions of the body. In the **cerebral cortex**, the thin layer of gray matter that constitutes the outer surface of the organ and that is made up of **billions of neurons**, sensations are made conscious, all voluntary activity is generated, and **higher mental processes**, involving thought, intelligence, memory, and language take place. Numerous interconnections between different areas of the cerebral cortex and **nerve nuclei** located inside the organ allow many functions to take place through mechanisms not yet well known. It is worth mentioning that, although there is still a lot to discover about the physiology of the brain, the areas of the cerebral cortex responsible for different functions have been located quite accurately. For example, it is known that voluntary movements originate in the **motor area** located in the precentral gyrus and that sensory stimuli are made conscious in the **sensory area** located in the postcentral gyrus.

CEREBRAL CONTROL IN A RIGHT-HANDED INDIVIDUAL

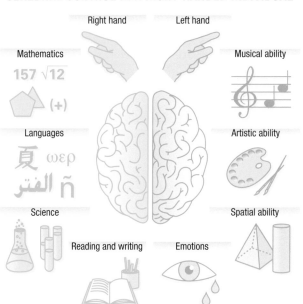

Right hand

Left hand

Mathematics

157 √12

(+)

Musical ability

Languages

夏 ωερ
ñ الفتر

Artistic ability

Science

Spatial ability

Reading and writing

Emotions

LATERALITY

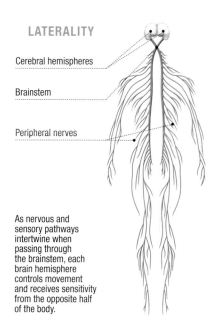

Cerebral hemispheres

Brainstem

Peripheral nerves

Each brain hemisphere, controls motility and senses on the opposite side of the body and has areas specialized in concrete mental functions. For example, in a right-handed individual, the right hemisphere is the location for musical and artistic abilities, spatial ability, and emotions, while the left hemisphere controls language, logic, and the analytical ability.

As nervous and sensory pathways intertwine when passing through the brainstem, each brain hemisphere controls movement and receives sensitivity from the opposite half of the body.

Introduction

A Perfect Machine

Skin

Digestive System

Nutrition

Respiratory System

Circulatory System and Blood

Nervous System

Musculoskeletal System

Urinary System

Endocrine System

Immune System

The Senses

Genetics

Reproductive System

Human Development

Index

MOTOR PATHWAYS

MOTOR PATHWAYS

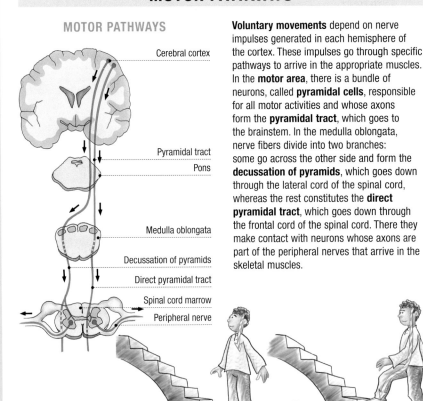

Cerebral cortex

Pyramidal tract

Pons

Medulla oblongata

Decussation of pyramids

Direct pyramidal tract

Spinal cord marrow

Peripheral nerve

Voluntary movements depend on nerve impulses generated in each hemisphere of the cortex. These impulses go through specific pathways to arrive in the appropriate muscles. In the **motor area**, there is a bundle of neurons, called **pyramidal cells**, responsible for all motor activities and whose axons form the **pyramidal tract**, which goes to the brainstem. In the medulla oblongata, nerve fibers divide into two branches: some go across the other side and form the **decussation of pyramids**, which goes down through the lateral cord of the spinal cord, whereas the rest constitutes the **direct pyramidal tract**, which goes down through the frontal cord of the spinal cord. There they make contact with neurons whose axons are part of the peripheral nerves that arrive in the skeletal muscles.

The spinal cord is an **extension of the brain**; it is a long cylinder inside the spinal column and from which the peripheral nerves arise. Actually, it constitutes a **communication path** between the brain and other brain structures, and the peripheral nervous system. In cross section, it can be observed that it has a central part in the shape of a butterfly made up of **gray matter**, which contains the bodies of several neurons. It is surrounded by a **white matter** area, made up of **bundles of nervous fibers** that travel the spinal cord: some **carry sensory information** from the periphery to the brain and others **transport motor impulses** in the opposite direction. All these fibers have a **specific order**, grouped in different cords or **fasciculi (funiculi)**: the ones carrying motor data, located in the front, and the ones taking different types of sensory information to the appropriate upper body structures in back.

SENSORY PATHWAYS

SENSORY PATHWAYS

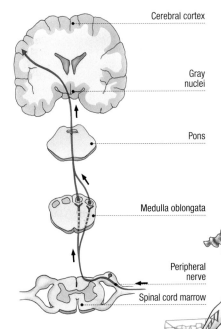

Cerebral cortex

Gray nuclei

Pons

Medulla oblongata

Peripheral nerve

Spinal cord marrow

The **sensory stimuli**, those from both outside the body (touch, pain, heat, cold, etc.) and inside the body (muscles, tendons, articulations, etc.) are detected by special **receptors** that trigger nerve impulses whose destination is the central nervous system. These impulses travel along the sensory nerve fibers, penetrate the spinal cord, and continue in an **ascending path** through specific cords according to the type of sensitivity they transmit until they reach certain brain structures. Thus, after several stops, they finally arrive in the **post-central gyrus** area of the cerebral cortex, where sensations are made conscious.

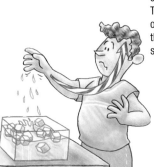

FUNCTION OF NERVES

A nerve is made up of **bundles of nervous fibers**, that is to say, axons of varied neurons that are surrounded by a wrapping of connective tissue. These fibers, and therefore the nerves, have a specific mission: they are in charge of **transmitting nerve impulses** from one place in the body to another, and they connect the central nervous system with the whole body. Nerve impulses transmitted by nerves respond to different kinds of signals. These signals can be either **sensory**, when they transmit impulses from sensory organs or from receptors inside the body toward the central nervous system, or **motor**, when they transmit orders from the central nervous system to the appropriate organs that can execute them, such as muscles or glands. There are nerves that are exclusively sensory or motor, but many are **mixed nerves** and they have both fibers that transmit sensory signals and fibers that spread motor signals.

STRUCTURE OF A NERVE

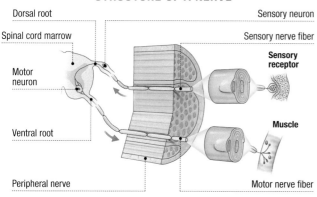

Dorsal root

Spinal cord marrow

Motor neuron

Ventral root

Peripheral nerve

Sensory neuron

Sensory nerve fiber

Sensory receptor

Muscle

Motor nerve fiber

SPINAL NERVES

From the spinal cord 31 pairs of **spinal nerves** or **nervi spinales** arise, which go through the vertebral foramina of the spine and later branch out, dividing into the nerves that arrive in all corners of the body: skin, muscles, internal abdominal glands, etc. They are **mixed nerves**, because they have both sensory fibers that transmit sensory stimuli to the spinal cord and motor fibers that transmit orders from the central nervous system to the effector organs.

SPINAL NERVES

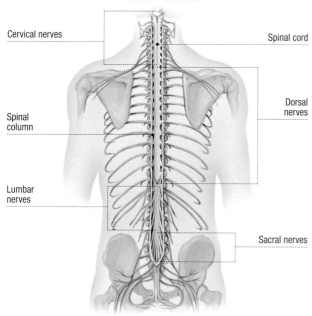

Cervical nerves

Spinal cord

Spinal column

Dorsal nerves

Lumbar nerves

Sacral nerves

CRANIAL NERVES

There are 12 nerves having their nucleus of origin or of destination in the brain and that emerge directly from the brain or the brainstem. They are called **cranial nerves**, and they arise from each side of the brain, and, although each one has a name, they are each designated with a Roman numeral from 1 (I) to 12 (XII). These nerves are very important, because some of them, such as the optic or auditory nerves, pick up sensory stimuli, whereas the others control the movements of the eyes or take part in the automatic regulation of the digestive, cardiac, and respiratory functions.

FUNCTION OF CRANIAL NERVES

Nerves	Name	Function
I	Olfactory	Transports smell impulses from nostrils to brain
II	Optic	Transports visual impulses from the retina to brain
III	Oculomotor	Takes part in the control of eye movement
IV	Trochlear	Takes part in the control of eye movement
V	Trigeminal	Provides for the sensitivity of the face and takes part in controlling chewing
VI	Abducens	Takes part in the control of eye movement
VII	Facial	Controls the movements of muscles in the face and carries taste sensations from the tongue to the brain
VIII	Acoustic or vestibulochear	Carries hearing impulses and stimuli that allow the control of balance in the inner ear to the brain
IX	Glosso-pharyngeal	Controls the movements of the muscles in the pharynx and carries taste sensations from the tongue to the brain
X	Vagus	Controls the movements of the pharynx and larynx, and takes part in the regulation of organs in the neck, thorax (heart, breathing), and the abdomen (digestive system)
XI	Accesory	Muscle movements of the neck
XII	Hypoglossal	Tongue movements

CRANIAL NERVES

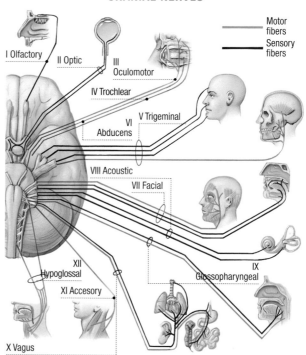

Motor fibers

Sensory fibers

I Olfactory

II Optic

III Oculomotor

IV Trochlear

V Trigeminal

VI Abducens

VIII Acoustic

VII Facial

XII Hypoglossal

XI Accesory

X Vagus

IX Glossopharyngeal

Introduction

A Perfect Machine

Skin

Digestive System

Nutrition

Respiratory System

Circulatory System and Blood

Nervous System

Musculoskeletal System

Urinary System

Endocrine System

Immune System

The Senses

Genetics

Reproductive System

Human Development

Index

REFLEXES

SIMPLE REFLEX ARC

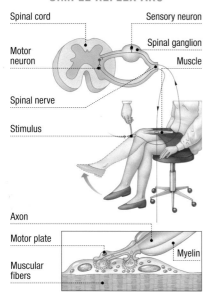

- Spinal cord
- Sensory neuron
- Motor neuron
- Spinal ganglion
- Muscle
- Spinal nerve
- Stimulus
- Axon
- Motor plate
- Myelin
- Muscular fibers

Unlike voluntary actions controlled by the brain, there are actions produced **automatically**, without intention, like when your finger gets pricked and you remove your hand immediately. These actions, in which the brain does not take part, are carried out by means of a circuit called **reflex action** in which only nerves and the spinal cord take part. In the simplest cases, such as the one in the example, the stimulus detected by skin receptors when your finger gets pricked travels through a **sensory neuron** to the spinal cord, and there it triggers a stimulus in a **motor neuron** that carries the impulse to the muscles in the hand, making it move away from the source of pain.

CONDITIONED REFLEXES

Simple reflexes are inherited and many of them can be observed from birth. Other reflexes you learn throughout life, and they require some participation from the cerebral cortex. Russian physiologist Ivan Petrovich Pavlov described conditioned reflexes toward the end of the nineteenth century. He observed that if he rang a bell each time he was going to feed his dog, the dog would start salivating upon hearing the bell. The dog's digestive system was getting ready to receive food when he recognized a stimulus that announced food. This kind of response, although with more complex mechanisms, is repeated frequently during our lives, and it is very important for the learning process.

The bath ritual, the milk bottle, and the cradle induce the baby to sleep.

THE AUTONOMIC NERVOUS SYSTEM

The **autonomic** or **vegetative nervous system** has the role of controlling the work of the internal abdominal organs, glands, blood vessels, and other organs so that they can respond appropriately and accordingly. This control is not done consciously, but automatically, that is to say without your will and without noticing. The autonomic nervous system is made up of several **nervous nuclei** of the brain, which send their messages through cranial nerves and fibers that come out of the spinal cord with the spinal nerves and form **ganglia** located next to the spinal column or near the organs they control. The autonomic nervous system has two distinct and complementary parts opposing each other to allow a delicate balance when the body adapts to the various everyday situations: the **sympathetic nervous system** and **the parasympathetic nervous system**. The former activates in situations of possible danger, the latter predominates in relaxed situations, at rest.

STRUCTURE OF THE AUTONOMOUS NERVOUS SYSTEM

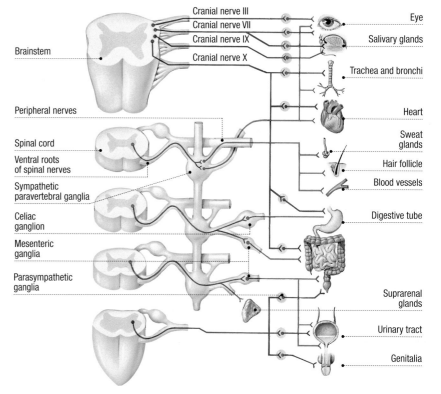

- Brainstem
- Cranial nerve III
- Cranial nerve VII
- Cranial nerve IX
- Cranial nerve X
- Peripheral nerves
- Spinal cord
- Ventral roots of spinal nerves
- Sympathetic paravertebral ganglia
- Celiac ganglion
- Mesenteric ganglia
- Parasympathetic ganglia
- Eye
- Salivary glands
- Trachea and bronchi
- Heart
- Sweat glands
- Hair follicle
- Blood vessels
- Digestive tube
- Suprarenal glands
- Urinary tract
- Genitalia

Introduction

A Perfect Machine

Skin

Digestive System

Nutrition

Respiratory System

Circulatory System and Blood

Nervous System

Musculoskeletal System

Urinary System

Endocrine System

Immune System

The Senses

Genetics

Reproductive System

Human Development

Index

ACTIONS OF THE AUTONOMIC NERVOUS SYSTEM

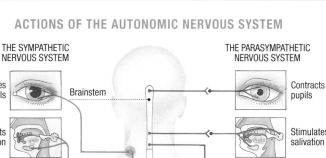

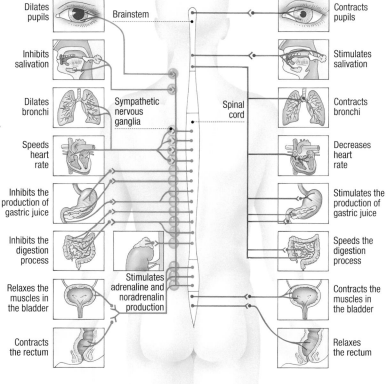

Predominance of the sympathetic nervous system

Predominance of the parasympathetic nervous system

The sympathetic nervous system activates in situations of possible danger and prepares us for fight or flight, while the parasympathetic nervous system is predominant during times of relaxation and peace.

THE SYMPATHETIC NERVOUS SYSTEM

- Dilates pupils
- Inhibits salivation
- Dilates bronchi
- Speeds heart rate
- Inhibits the production of gastric juice
- Inhibits the digestion process
- Relaxes the muscles in the bladder
- Contracts the rectum

Brainstem
Sympathetic nervous ganglia
Stimulates adrenaline and noradrenalin production

Spinal cord

THE PARASYMPATHETIC NERVOUS SYSTEM

- Contracts pupils
- Stimulates salivation
- Contracts bronchi
- Decreases heart rate
- Stimulates the production of gastric juice
- Speeds the digestion process
- Contracts the muscles in the bladder
- Relaxes the rectum

ADRENALINE RUSH: FIGHT OR FLIGHT

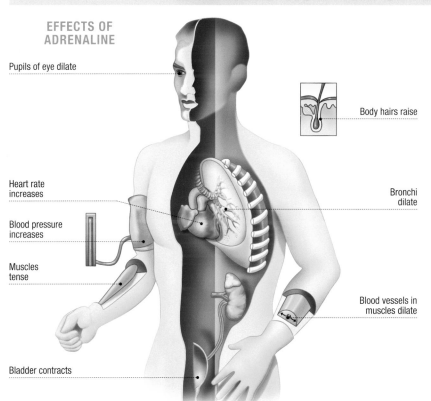

EFFECTS OF ADRENALINE

- Pupils of eye dilate
- Heart rate increases
- Blood pressure increases
- Muscles tense
- Bladder contracts
- Body hairs raise
- Bronchi dilate
- Blood vessels in muscles dilate

When we face a stressful situation, a situation that scares us, or one that requires an immediate response, the sympathetic nervous system goes into action, making, in only a few seconds, several modifications in the functioning of the body so that we are able to solve the problem in a better way. It has a very special behavior: in view of danger, it stimulates the **adrenal glands** so that they can release a hormone called **adrenaline** into the blood stream, which then goes throughout the body. Different organs have **specific receptors** for adrenaline that respond to the stimulus immediately: the heart beats faster, muscles tense up…

Reflexes are essential to ensure the survival of an individual, protecting from external attacks and maintaining the vital functions of the body.

THE MUSCULOSKELETAL SYSTEM

The musculoskeletal system is made up of several structures that work harmoniously and in coordination so that we can move and make all the gestures we want to make. **Bones** constitute the **framework** of the body, **joints** allow the **movement** in different parts of the body, and **muscles** provide the necessary **strength** to realize the movements.

COMPONENTS OF THE MUSCULOSKELETAL SYSTEM

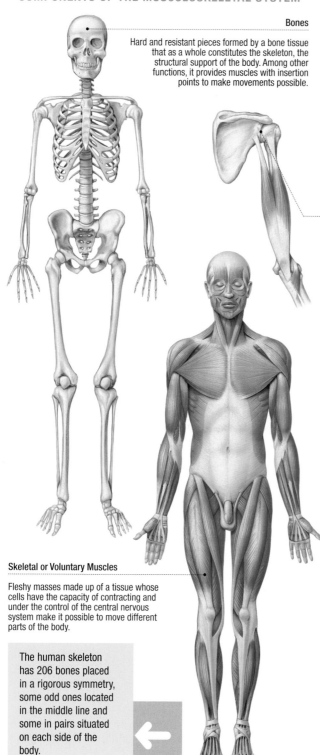

Bones

Hard and resistant pieces formed by a bone tissue that as a whole constitutes the skeleton, the structural support of the body. Among other functions, it provides muscles with insertion points to make movements possible.

Joints

A set of structures that constitute the connecting points with bones, some fixed and some mobile, allowing different types of movements.

Skeletal or Voluntary Muscles

Fleshy masses made up of a tissue whose cells have the capacity of contracting and under the control of the central nervous system make it possible to move different parts of the body.

The human skeleton has 206 bones placed in a rigorous symmetry, some odd ones located in the middle line and some in pairs situated on each side of the body.

LEVER SYSTEM

The different structures forming the musculoskeletal system work, in a sense, like a lever system. The bones, which are the **rigid segments**, correspond to the levers, whereas joints represent the **fulcrums**, and the muscles are in charge of generating and applying the strength that produces movement. So, when a muscle contracts, it moves the bones where it is inserted and, depending on the joint that joins them, causes a certain movement. The different muscles **work together** coordinated by the central nervous system and produce **body movements** that we make voluntarily and, in short, allows us to move from one place to another.

FUNCTIONS OF BONES

The bones that make up the skeleton have as their most important role locomotion, but they also have other functions:

Support. The skeleton is the body's framework, and it is the basis to which all muscles and tendons are connected.

Protection. Some components of the skeleton protect certain parts of the body, especially soft and vulnerable organs, from blows and other external attacks.

Mineral deposit. The organic reservoir of minerals, such as calcium and phosphorus, corresponds mainly to the content in the bones.

Blood production. Blood cells are formed in the bone marrow inside some bones. These cells then go into the blood stream as red cells, white cells, and platelets.

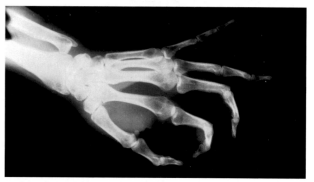

Through X-ray, possible fractures or deformities in bones can be checked.

BONE TISSUE ACTIVITY

Bones are not, as sometimes thought, lifeless. They are made up of **living tissue** that, although it may not seem like it, is in **constant activity**. Bone tissue is made up of an **organic matrix** having cells, collagen fibers, and an **amorphous substance**, which constitutes the framework over which minerals such as calcium and phosphorus are deposited, giving bones their characteristic toughness. Three types of specialized cells can be identified in this particular tissue: **osteoblasts**, **osteocytes**,

and **osteoclasts**. Osteoblasts are in charge of producing **bone material**, where minerals are deposited. Osteocytes are actually inactive osteoblasts trapped within bone material. Osteoclasts destroy and reabsorb worn bone tissue. Due to the coordinated activity and the delicate balance of all cells, bone tissue is renewed under the control of several hormones, and also, bones reform with the passage of time.

COMPONENTS OF BONE TISSUE

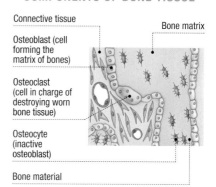

Connective tissue

Bone matrix

Osteoblast (cell forming the matrix of bones)

Osteoclast (cell in charge of destroying worn bone tissue)

Osteocyte (inactive osteoblast)

Bone material

DIAGRAM OF A BONE SECTION

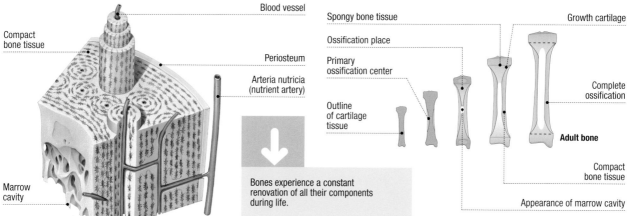

Blood vessel

Compact bone tissue

Periosteum

Arteria nutricia (nutrient artery)

Marrow cavity

OSSIFICATION PROCESS OF A LONG BONE

Spongy bone tissue

Ossification place

Primary ossification center

Outline of cartilage tissue

Growth cartilage

Complete ossification

Adult bone

Compact bone tissue

Appearance of marrow cavity

Bones experience a constant renovation of all their components during life.

BONE STRUCTURE

Bone tissue presents a **complex structure**. The bone material produced by osteoblasts, and on top of which minerals are deposited, must be placed in such a way that allows the passage of blood vessels carrying cell nutrients and construction material inside the bone. In the external part of the bone, surrounded by a layer of resistant tissue called **periosteum**, bone plates (lamellae) are **concentric**, and they are arranged around a **central canal** through which a blood vessel travels. Several canaliculi go through the lamellae, allowing the canal's ramifications to go through them. This unit is called the **Haversian system**. The lamellae are closely and tightly connected to each other, forming a hard mass, which provides the bone with resistance. This is called **compact bone tissue**. But inside the bone, the lamellae are arranged in **irregular trabeculae**, which leave free spaces in between, forming a **spongy bone tissue**. This tissue is less dense, has a porous appearance, and contains bone marrow, which is in charge of making blood.

BONE GROWTH

Bone formation starts with gestation, but it takes a long time to complete. At first, the skeleton is made up of **cartilaginous tissue**, which forms a flexible and elastic mold of all bones, because it does not have minerals. This tissue is progressively replaced by harder and more resistant bone tissue by means of a process called **ossification**. During this process, **ossification centers** appear in the thickness of the cartilage, from where active bone cells form the organic bone matrix, which later on will be mineralized. Primary ossification centers appear during fetal life, but throughout childhood other ossification centers appear, which allow the bone to grow in length and thickness. There is something particular about long bones, because in the place where the shaft of a long bone (diaphysis) meets the ends of the long bones (epiphysis), there are growth cartilages, from which bone

stretching occurs during childhood. These areas only ossify in puberty, under the influence of hormones, and this determines the end of development and the final size of the individual.

EVOLUTION OF BONE MASS ACCORDING TO AGE

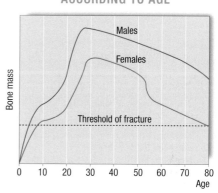

Males

Females

Threshold of fracture

Bone mass

0 10 20 30 40 50 60 70 80

Age

Bone mass increases progressively during childhood, and it has a greater increase in adolescence. After age 30, it starts to decrease, although under normal conditions, bones continue being tough until old age.

The skeleton has 99% of the calcium and 85% of the phosphorus in the body.

MUSCLES

Muscles can contract and relax; they can **modify their length**, allowing certain mechanical effects. The human body has different kinds of muscles performing different functions. Some are **smooth muscles**, controlled by the autonomic nervous system and whose actions do not depend on our will. This type of muscle can be found in most of the internal organs in the abdomen. Smooth muscles allow the changes in diameter of the arteries, the movements in the stomach and the intestine, and the emptying of the bladder. Others are called **striated muscles**, because if observed under the electron microscope, they show characteristic striations. A very special one is the **cardiac muscle** whose action is involuntary and automatic. The rest of the muscles are **skeletal striated muscles**, also called **somatic** or **voluntary**, because the brain controls them; they contract or relax according to our will. These are the muscles that belong to the locomotor system and that make the body move.

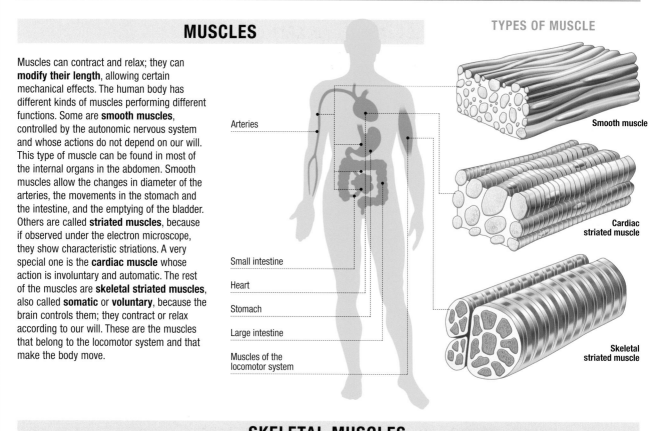

Arteries

Small intestine

Heart

Stomach

Large intestine

Muscles of the locomotor system

Smooth muscle

Cardiac striated muscle

Skeletal striated muscle

SKELETAL MUSCLES

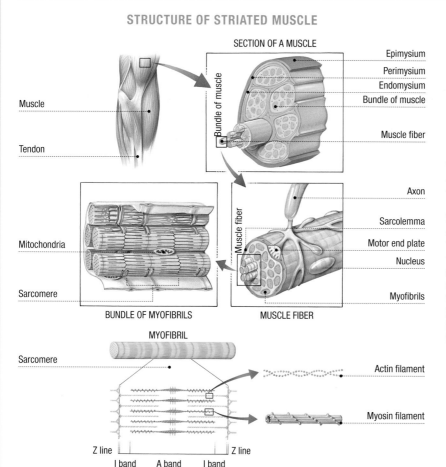

SECTION OF A MUSCLE

Muscle

Tendon

Bundle of muscle

Epimysium
Perimysium
Endomysium
Bundle of muscle

Muscle fiber

Mitochondria

Sarcomere

BUNDLE OF MYOFIBRILS

Muscle fiber

Axon

Sarcolemma

Motor end plate

Nucleus

Myofibrils

MUSCLE FIBER

MYOFIBRIL

Sarcomere

Actin filament

Myosin filament

Z line   Z line
I band   A band   I band

The muscles in the locomotor system are basically made up of elongated cells called **muscle fibers** grouped in **bundles** or **fascicles** and wrapped by sheaths of connective tissue. Each muscle fiber has hundreds or thousands of very thin **myofibrils**, which lie along the cell. Thanks to them, muscles can contract and relax. These myofibrils are the ones having the **striations** that are so characteristic and that give their name to striated muscles. Striations are transverse segments, of various thicknesses that follow a well-defined pattern and allow the identification of **sarcomeres**, functional units in the muscle. Each sarcomere is delimited on each side by a dark striation, a **Z line**, while inside it has a darker, wider band, an **A band**, and two lighter bands, **I bands**. These bands coincide with the presence of filaments from two types of protein, **myosin** and **actin**, arranged longitudinally inside the sarcomere. **Myosin filaments**, which are thicker, occupy the center and give the A band its dark color. **Actin filaments**, which are thinner, penetrate the Z lines and give I bands their lighter color.

CONTRACTION AND RELAXATION OF MUSCLES

Muscles contract according to the orders from the central nervous system. Neuron extensions reach the muscle fibers and transmit the timely **motor impulses**, which determine the shortening of the sarcomeres. In each sarcomere, myosin and actin filaments alternate, and they are partially tied at rest, when the muscle is relaxed. When a nerve impulse is received, it generates the **action potential** that causes the actin filaments to slide in between the myosin filaments decreasing the distance between Z lines and shortening the sarcomere. Myofibrils also shorten, and the muscle fibers that are stimulated contract. When the nerve stimulus stops, actin filaments move in the opposite direction, sarcomeres lengthen, and muscle fibers regain their previous dimensions, causing the muscle to relax.

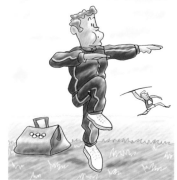

The human body has 640 different muscles, each with its own function.

MUSCLE CONTRACTION AND MUSCLE RELAXATION MECHANISM

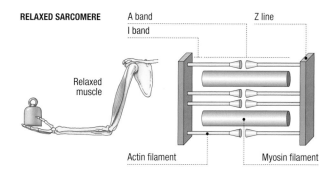

RELAXED SARCOMERE

A band
I band
Z line

Relaxed muscle

Actin filament
Myosin filament

CONTRACTED SARCOMERE

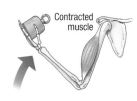

Contracted muscle

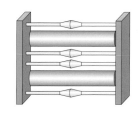

MUSCLE METABOLISM

Muscles need **energy** to be able to contract. Like other cells in the body, muscle fibers obtain energy from the oxygen-dependent combustion of glucose, called **aerobic metabolism**. The waste products of this combustion are carbon dioxide molecules that are later transported in the blood to the lungs for their elimination. But striated muscle cells have a special energy resource that allows them to perform intense activity before the blood can supply enough oxygen, and this is **anaerobic metabolism**. This metabolism generates a residue of molecules of lactic acid. This mechanism is only efficient for a short time, at most 20 or 30 seconds, although the amount of energy that it provides to the muscle is high. It is also responsible for fatigue, because the buildup of lactic acid causes intense tiredness, and it also causes that typical "stiffness" that appears after unusual exercise. To avoid this, it is important to do warm-up exercises before physical activity, because blood circulation in the muscles increases and so does the oxygen supply.

TYPES OF MUSCLE METABOLISM

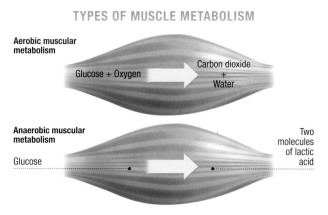

Aerobic muscular metabolism

Glucose + Oxygen → Carbon dioxide + Water

Anaerobic muscular metabolism

Glucose → Two molecules of lactic acid

MOVEMENT COORDINATION

Muscles are attached to bones or to other more or less solid-body structures directly or by means of fiber bands called **tendons**. Thereby, there is movement of a part of the skeleton. In order to move, different muscles must coordinate perfectly, because movement is dependent on the activity of **muscle groups** made up of muscles of opposite action. When a movement is made, not only **agonist** muscles are involved, but also **synergetic** and **antagonist** muscles. Agonist muscles are the most active and the most important, synergetic muscles give support, and antagonist muscles must relax to allow movement. For example, when the forearm flexes over the arm, the biceps contracts and the triceps relaxes, whereas to extend the forearm exactly the opposite has to happen. If antagonist and agonist muscles contract at the same time, there would be no movement.

AGONIST AND ANTAGONIST MUSCLES

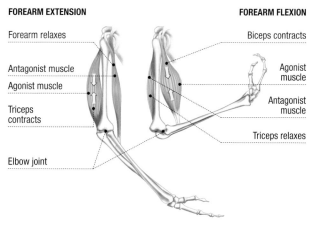

FOREARM EXTENSION

Forearm relaxes

Antagonist muscle

Agonist muscle

Triceps contracts

Elbow joint

FOREARM FLEXION

Biceps contracts

Agonist muscle

Antagonist muscle

Triceps relaxes

JOINTS

Joints are the **connection points** between the various parts of the skeleton. They are made up of the contact surface of two or more bones and a series of elements that guarantee such a union and provide stability. Actually, some joints are immovable and are named **synarthroses**. They are the solid union of two or more bones, and their main role is to provide protection to the organs they cover, such as the joints of the skull that protect the brain. There are also some slightly mobile joints called **amphiarthroses**. The bone surfaces that form part of this type of joint are not directly joined but are separated by a fibrous cartilage that only allows slight movement. An example is the joints in the vertebrae of the spine, separated by a intervertebral disk. Finally, **movable joints** are called **diarthroses** and allow a wide range of movement, such as joints in shoulders, hips, or elbows. These are the basic components of the locomotor system, which allow us to move the various parts of the body.

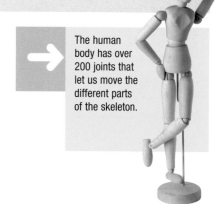

The human body has over 200 joints that let us move the different parts of the skeleton.

STRUCTURE OF A SIMPLE MOVABLE JOINT

Ligaments

Fibrous bands that provide the joint with more stability

Synovial membrane

Tissue that covers the inside of the joint capsule and is in charge of making synovial fluid

Articular cartilage

Thin band of tissue, resistant and elastic, that covers the bone ends and prevents the bones from rubbing directly when moving, to avoid wear and tear

Joint capsule

Fibrous and resistant membrane enclosing the joint that is firmly inserted in the bones it joins

Synovial Fluid

Yellowish and viscous fluid that fills the joint, whose role is to lubricate the contact surfaces and to nourish articular cartilages

TYPES OF MOVABLE JOINTS

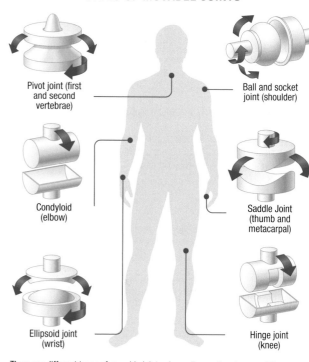

Pivot joint (first and second vertebrae)

Ball and socket joint (shoulder)

Condyloid (elbow)

Saddle Joint (thumb and metacarpal)

Ellipsoid joint (wrist)

Hinge joint (knee)

There are different types of movable joints, depending on the shape and the way connecting bone segments fit; each one of them allows some specific movements.

SHOULDER MOVEMENTS

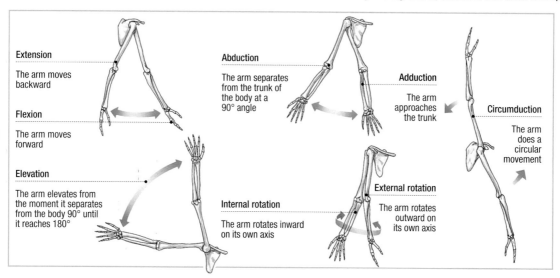

Extension

The arm moves backward

Flexion

The arm moves forward

Elevation

The arm elevates from the moment it separates from the body 90° until it reaches 180°

Abduction

The arm separates from the trunk of the body at a 90° angle

Adduction

The arm approaches the trunk

Internal rotation

The arm rotates inward on its own axis

External rotation

The arm rotates outward on its own axis

Circumduction

The arm does a circular movement

The shoulder has the most movable joint, scapulohumeral, because it provides a wide range of arm movements, each with a different name.

WALKING MECHANICS

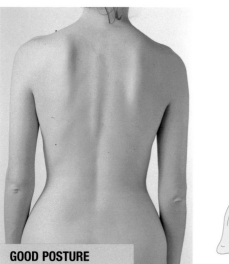

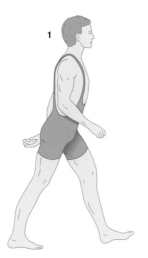

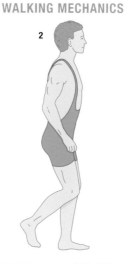

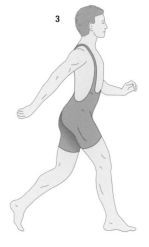

GOOD POSTURE

The spine is the **axis of the skeleton** and, besides supporting a good part of the total body weight, is usually under much strain in everyday life. The ligaments and muscles that join the vertebrae provide the spine with some stability. Sometimes that is not enough, especially in two areas that suffer greater stress: **the neck area** and **the lumbar area**. The neck area is responsible for all head movements and many times assumes a poor posture, for example, when reading or doing manual tasks. The lumbar region suffers the most demands. Many activities and postures place an exaggerated stress on one or another part of the spine and favor **deviations** of the spine or are the source of **back pain**. That is why it is important to be aware of the characteristics of the spine and to know how we can subject it to much harm during the day. It is important to try to keep the back straight and to avoid sudden gestures, forced actions, and all those positions that curve or twist the back.

1. The left heel touches the ground, then you put the weight on the sole of the foot; this goes together with a swinging movement of the right arm.
2. When the left foot bears all the weight of the body, the heel of the right foot goes up, leaving the tip and then lifting the whole foot.
3. The right foot moves forward, and it rests on the ground, the left arm has a swinging motion.

Walking, in humans, is done on two feet in a coordinated and rhythmic sequence of movements alternating elevation and forward motion of the foot before lifting the other foot. This is accompanied by a swinging motion of the arms.

ADVICE TO PREVENT BACK PAIN

Not advisable	Advisable	Not advisable	Advisable
To sleep on a soft mattress with a flexible base of the bed	To sleep on a mattress that is not too soft with a wooden bed base	To carry a heavy weight far from the body	To carry a heavy weight close to the body
To sleep on your stomach	To sleep on the side	To carry a lot of weight in one arm	To distribute the weight in both arms
To lift your upper body suddenly while keeping the legs straight in order to get up from bed	To roll to the edge of the bed and place the legs out before getting up	To push a heavy object while facing it	To push a heavy object by using your back to push
To reach up to get an object located above	To step on a stool to reach an object located up high	To sit with a spine inclined forward	To sit with a straight back and both feet on the ground
To bend at the waist to pick up a heavy weight	To bend the knees to pick up a heavy weight	To sit on sofas too soft or sit without bending your knees	To sit on sofas with good back support and arm rests

THE URINARY SYSTEM

The urinary system is in charge of **filtering the blood**, which is constantly circulating in the body, to **regulate its composition**. But it also filters the blood with the main purpose of expelling, through urine, excess water, salts, toxic products, and **metabolic residues** whose collection in the body could be harmful.

COMPONENTS OF THE URINARY SYSTEM

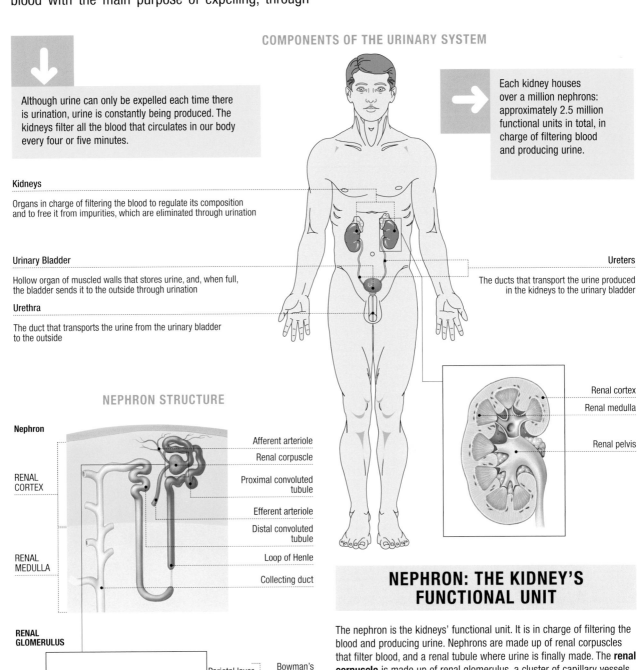

Although urine can only be expelled each time there is urination, urine is constantly being produced. The kidneys filter all the blood that circulates in our body every four or five minutes.

Each kidney houses over a million nephrons: approximately 2.5 million functional units in total, in charge of filtering blood and producing urine.

Kidneys

Organs in charge of filtering the blood to regulate its composition and to free it from impurities, which are eliminated through urination

Urinary Bladder

Hollow organ of muscled walls that stores urine, and, when full, the bladder sends it to the outside through urination

Urethra

The duct that transports the urine from the urinary bladder to the outside

Ureters

The ducts that transport the urine produced in the kidneys to the urinary bladder

Renal cortex
Renal medulla
Renal pelvis

NEPHRON STRUCTURE

Nephron

RENAL CORTEX

RENAL MEDULLA

Afferent arteriole
Renal corpuscle
Proximal convoluted tubule
Efferent arteriole
Distal convoluted tubule
Loop of Henle
Collecting duct

RENAL GLOMERULUS

Parietal layer
Visceral layer
Bowman's capsule
Renal tubule
Urinary space
Glomerular capillaries

NEPHRON: THE KIDNEY'S FUNCTIONAL UNIT

The nephron is the kidneys' functional unit. It is in charge of filtering the blood and producing urine. Nephrons are made up of renal corpuscles that filter blood, and a renal tubule where urine is finally made. The **renal corpuscle** is made up of renal glomerulus, a cluster of capillary vessels, and it is surrounded by a double membrane in the shape of a funnel called **Bowman's capsule**, which is a continuation of the renal tubule. The glomerulus corresponds to the branches of the **afferent arteriole**, which take blood to the renal corpuscle; these later join to form the **efferent arteriole** through which the already filtered blood comes out. In between the two layers of Bowman's capsule, there is a minute fissure, the **urinary space**, where the product of the glomerural filtration is poured. The continuation of this capsule, the **renal tubule**, is in charge of processing the glomerural product to make urine, which finally goes to a **collecting duct**, which collects the urine coming from various nephrons and takes it to the urinary ducts.

Introduction

A Perfect Machine

Skin

Digestive System

Nutrition

Respiratory System

Circulatory System and Blood

Nervous System

Musculoskeletal System

Urinary System

Endocrine System

Immune System

The Senses

Genetics

Reproductive System

Human Development

Index

PRESSURE INVOLVED IN GLOMERURAL FILTRATION

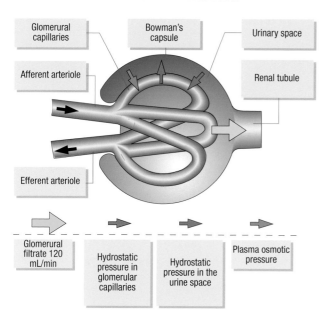

Glomerural capillaries

Bowman's capsule

Urinary space

Afferent arteriole

Renal tubule

Efferent arteriole

Glomerural filtrate 120 mL/min

Hydrostatic pressure in glomerular capillaries

Hydrostatic pressure in the urine space

Plasma osmotic pressure

SIMULATION OF THE PROCESS OF GLOMERULAR FILTRATION

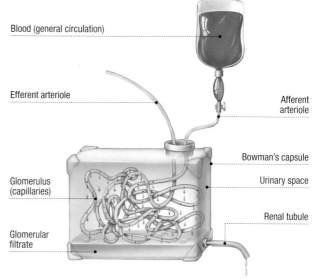

Blood (general circulation)

Efferent arteriole

Afferent arteriole

Bowman's capsule

Urinary space

Glomerulus (capillaries)

Renal tubule

Glomerular filtrate

BLOOD FILTRATION

The first step in the **formation of urine** corresponds to a filtration process in which part of the plasma goes through small pores present in the walls of the glomerular capillaries and goes to the urinary place between the two layers of Bowman's capsule to continue its path through the renal tubule. The filtration process is a **passive process** in which two opposite forces are involved: **hydrostatic pressure**, the pressure of the liquid in each compartment, and **plasma osmotic pressure**, the water attraction power that proteins present in the plasma have and that cannot go through the pores of the walls of the glomerulus capillaries due to their size. A **filtration pressure** results from the interaction of forces, which means the passage of water and of various substances of small size dissolved in the plasma inside the urine space.

DOPING IS A DANGEROUS AND UNFAIR PRACTICE

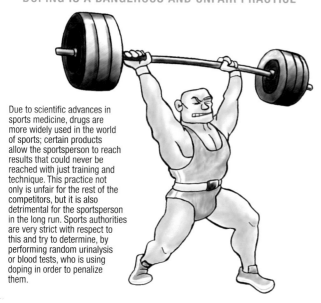

Due to scientific advances in sports medicine, drugs are more widely used in the world of sports; certain products allow the sportsperson to reach results that could never be reached with just training and technique. This practice not only is unfair for the rest of the competitors, but it is also detrimental for the sportsperson in the long run. Sports authorities are very strict with respect to this and try to determine, by performing random urinalysis or blood tests, who is using doping in order to penalize them.

URINE FORMATION

Glomerular filtrate, when passing through the renal tubules, changes dramatically. Most of the water and various substances are **reabsorbed**; they go to the adjacent capillary vessels and back into the bloodstream. Other substances not filtered in the glomerulus are **secreted** in the opposite direction, which means they go from the blood in the nearby capillaries into the tubule. Due to that, the 180 liters a day of glomerular filtrate turns into only 1.5-2 liters of urine. The body recovers **useful substances** that have been filtered in the glomerulus and gets rid of others to keep an adequate physical and chemical balance of the internal environment. Some steps in this process are performed by **passive transport mechanisms**, because some substances tend to equalize their concentration in both compartments, whereas others are performed by **active transport mechanisms** that determine the passage of substances in the opposite direction to that of passive transport. Thus the glomerular filtrate changes as it moves through the renal tubules; a great amount of the filtered water is reabsorbed, as are other useful substances for the body, such as glucose, amino acids, phosphates, and bicarbonate.

URINALYSIS

The **composition of urine** has a direct relationship with the composition of blood in our body. It seems logical that the analysis of urine reflects the **functioning of the body**. It is not surprising, then, that urinalysis has become a test requested by many physicians and that it constitutes a key part of any **medical checkup**. It is easy to do and is without major discomfort; it aids in the **evaluation** of kidney activity and in the **diagnosis** of possible alterations of various organs.

REGULATION OF URINE VOLUME

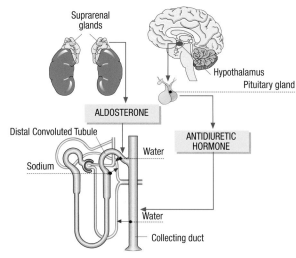

Suprarenal glands

Hypothalamus

Pituitary gland

ALDOSTERONE

Distal Convoluted Tubule

Sodium

Water

ANTIDIURETIC HORMONE

Water

Collecting duct

CONTROL OF KIDNEY FUNCTION

The volume of urine produced by the kidneys is not uniform, because it varies according to body needs and is related to the amount of water taken in with drink and food. Most of the water filtered in the glomerulus is reabsorbed in the initial part of the renal tubules and goes back into the blood. Another important amount is reabsorbed in the distal area and especially in the collecting pump under the influence of two hormones: **aldosterone** and **antidiuretic hormone**. The former is secreted by the adrenal glands acting in the distal convoluted tubule and causes an increase in sodium and water reabsorption, whereas the latter is made in the hypothalamus and is secreted by the pituitary, acting especially in the collecting duct and increasing water permeability, thus increasing its reabsorption. Then, if we drink a little, little urine will be made, but if we drink a lot, we will urinate much more.

THE PROCEDURE OF PERITONEAL DIALYSIS

Dialysis solution

Infusion tube

Drainage tube

Drainage bag

DIAGRAM OF HEMODIALYSIS

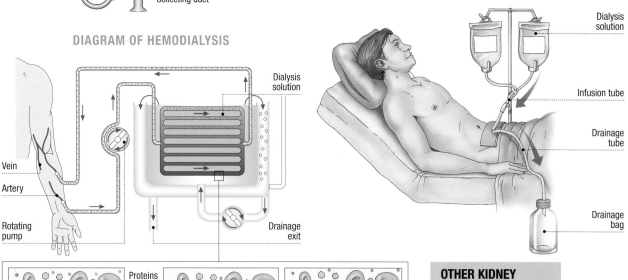

Dialysis solution

Vein

Artery

Rotating pump

Drainage exit

Proteins

Blood

Red cells

Semipermeable membrane

Dialysis solution

Waste products

The substances that can go through pores of the membrane go to the dialysis solution.

A balance is accomplished when the concentrations on both sides of the membrane are equal.

HEMODIALYSIS: THE ARTIFICIAL KIDNEY

If kidney activity fails, various organic disorders appear and life is threatened. Human inventiveness has created a method to substitute renal activity, even if only partially. **Dialysis** is a technique that allows the elimination of waste products in blood and the excess fluid in the body when kidneys are no longer able to do it. The technique is based on the use of **semi-permeable membranes**, which allow the free passage of fluids; but, only small particles can go through, holding back bigger ones, just like the renal

glomerulus does. Because the substances present in the solutions separated by a semipermeable membrane tend to balance their concentrations on both sides, it is possible to **purify blood**, making it circulate right next to a membrane with these characteristics if, on the other side, a solution of special composition is placed, called **dialysate**. Waste products whose concentration is higher in the blood will go through the membrane and will go into the dialysate in the right amount to achieve a balance.

OTHER KIDNEY FUNCTIONS

The kidneys, besides making urine, perform other important functions. On the one hand, they participate in the **regulation** of the **blood pressure**. When the volume of circulating blood and the renal blood flow decrease, the kidneys release substances that cause a contraction of the blood vessels and stimulate the suprarenal glands to make them increase their production of the hormone, called aldosterone. This hormone favors sodium and water reabsorption in the renal tubules, indirectly causing an increase in the blood pressure. On the other hand, it contributes to the **production of red cells** in the blood. When the blood circulating in the kidneys has a small concentration of oxygen, the kidneys release a substance that, after passing through the liver, turns into **erythropoietin**, a hormone that stimulates the production of erythrocytes in the bone marrow.

URINATION MECHANISM

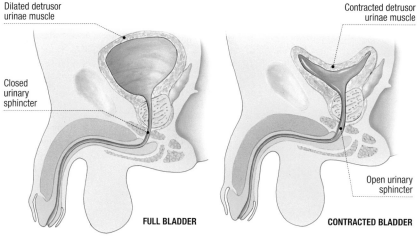

Dilated detrusor urinae muscle

Closed urinary sphincter

FULL BLADDER

Contracted detrusor urinae muscle

Open urinary sphincter

CONTRACTED BLADDER

Introduction

A Perfect Machine

Skin

Digestive System

Nutrition

Respiratory System

Circulatory System and Blood

Nervous System

Musculoskeletal System

Urinary System

Endocrine System

Immune System

The Senses

Genetics

Reproductive System

Human Development

Index

URINATION

The urine produced endlessly in the kidneys goes to the **ureters**, reaching the urinary bladder, where it is stored. This storage place is only temporary, because the capacity of the bladder has a limit and when this limit is exceeded, urine is expelled out through the **urethra** due to the **urination mechanism**. This mechanism relies on a type of muscle valve located at the bladder's end that allows the urethra to remain closed. As a matter of fact, this valve, the **urinary sphincter**, is formed by two structures, each constituting a barrier for the passage of urine. The **internal urethral sphincter** is located at the site where the bladder connects with the urethra, and the **external urethral sphincter** is located in the middle section of the urethra. The former works automatically, but the latter, up to a certain point, can be controlled at will; this makes it possible to "hold" the urine until you find the right moment to eliminate it in appropriate conditions.

URINATION CONTROL

Elimination is produced due to an **automatic reflex** that is triggered when the bladder walls distend over a certain limit. When this happens, some nerve receptors located on the bladder walls send a signal that reaches the **micturation center** located in the spinal cord, which responds, sending motor impulses that reach the muscle layer of the bladder walls. That is when the **detrusor muscle**, which forms part of the bladder wall, contracts and at the same time the internal urethral sphincter opens allowing the urine out into the urethra. However, so that the urine is eliminated, it is necessary that the external urethral sphincter, which is under the control of will, relax. Under normal conditions, this happens only when the brain, after receiving stimuli indicating that the bladder is full, decides that the necessary conditions are present to produce elimination.

URINATION REFLEX

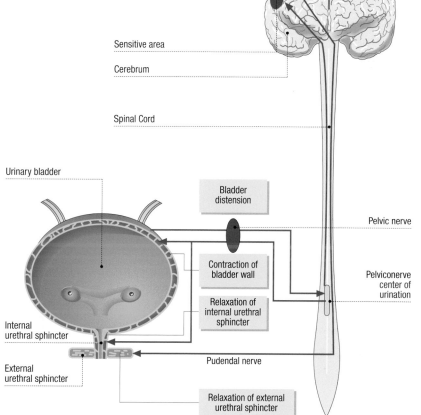

Motor area

Sensitive area

Cerebrum

Spinal Cord

Urinary bladder

Bladder distension

Contraction of bladder wall

Relaxation of internal urethral sphincter

Internal urethral sphincter

External urethral sphincter

Pelvic nerve

Pelviconerve center of urination

Pudendal nerve

Relaxation of external urethral sphincter

WETTING THE BED

Many older children wet the bed at night. Some of them do it once in a while, whereas others do it many times. This is known as **enuresis**, and it is the involuntary elimination of urine during the time of rest, at night, at an age when the person should control the urinary sphincter (over the age of four or five). Actually, it is a very common problem; and, although in a few cases, it can be attributed to a physical problem in the urinary system, it generally is a consequence of a delay in the learning process of how to control sphincters.

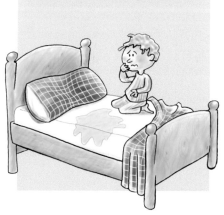

THE ENDOCRINE SYSTEM

The endocrine system is in charge of **regulating** the body's functioning by means of **hormones**. Hormones are substances produced by a series of **glands of internal secretion**, and, once in the blood, they are transported to every part of the body. Hormones act as chemical **messengers** to control the activity, metabolism, growth, and development of the various tissues and organs.

A REAL ORGANIC SYSTEM

Unlike other organic systems, such as the digestive or urinary systems, whose components have a direct anatomical relationship, the endocrine system is made up of various **glands of internal secretion** located in different parts of the body, far from one another and without any anatomical continuation. However, these glands constitute a true organic system, because their activity is **closely related**. For example, some of them depend on either the **stimulation** or **inhibition** of other hormones produced by different glands. Many hormones produced in the various endocrine glands have actions that are either similar or opposite, and, therefore, the overall effect depends on a **delicate balance** of the whole.

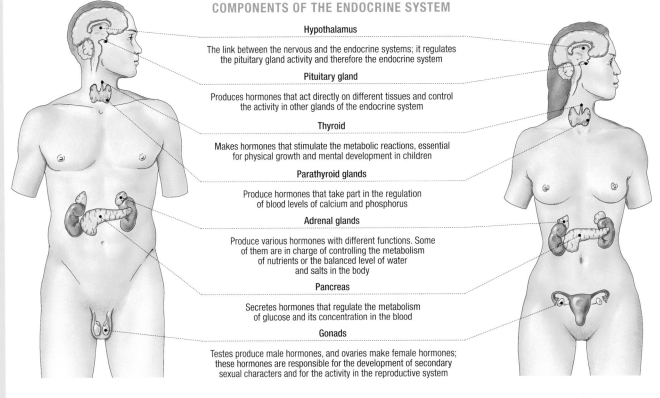

COMPONENTS OF THE ENDOCRINE SYSTEM

Hypothalamus
The link between the nervous and the endocrine systems; it regulates the pituitary gland activity and therefore the endocrine system

Pituitary gland
Produces hormones that act directly on different tissues and control the activity in other glands of the endocrine system

Thyroid
Makes hormones that stimulate the metabolic reactions, essential for physical growth and mental development in children

Parathyroid glands
Produce hormones that take part in the regulation of blood levels of calcium and phosphorus

Adrenal glands
Produce various hormones with different functions. Some of them are in charge of controlling the metabolism of nutrients or the balanced level of water and salts in the body

Pancreas
Secretes hormones that regulate the metabolism of glucose and its concentration in the blood

Gonads
Testes produce male hormones, and ovaries make female hormones; these hormones are responsible for the development of secondary sexual characters and for the activity in the reproductive system

FEEDBACK MECHANISM

The activity of the endocrine system is subject to **multiple influences**, because it must adapt to the **ever-changing needs** of the body. As a matter of fact, the hypothalamus, which is also part of the nervous system, receives numerous **stimuli** from outside and from the internal environment. But the endocrine system also has a particular **control mechanism** of hormonal secretions, called **feedback**. In the case of some hormones, their own blood levels are a determinant factor to increase or to decrease their production. So, when the blood concentration of a hormone decreases below certain ranges, the hypothalamus and the pituitary gland detect this and act upon the gland in charge of producing it to cause it to increase its secretion. That is **positive feedback**. And when the blood levels of a hormone exceeds certain ranges, the hypothalamus and the pituitary gland register this fact and stop stimulating the producing gland, making it reduce its activity. This is **negative feedback**. This mechanism ensures that each hormone circulates in blood in the amount needed to accomplish its task.

FEEDBACK MECHANISM
IN HORMONAL SECRETION

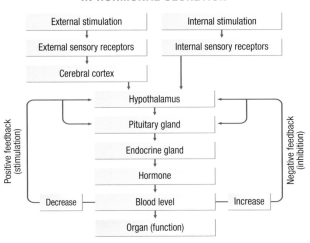

FUNCTIONS OF THE HYPOTHALAMUS

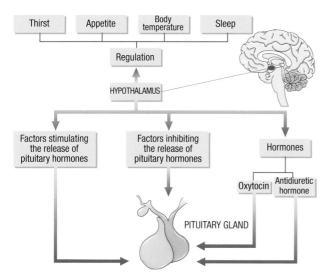

THE HYPOTHALAMUS, THE "BOSS" OF THE ENDOCRINE SYSTEM

The hypothalamus has varied activities, because it houses **nerve centers** that direct such important things as thirst, the appetite, body temperature, and sleep. It is also involved in the regulation of heart rate and blood pressure. However, this small structure located in a **privileged situation**, at the base of the cerebrum, is connected to different areas of the nervous system and therefore is able to receive many stimuli, physical and mental. It has another important function: its role as a **regulator of the endocrine system**. The hypothalamus produces many **hormonal factors** that either stimulate or inhibit the production of hormones by the pituitary gland, which regulates the endocrine system through its secretions. Thus, the hypothalamus is the structure that really **controls** the activity of the internal glands and adapts its functioning to the ever-changing needs of the body according to the data it gets from the internal environment and from outside. Besides, it also produces two hormones, oxytocin and the antidiuretic hormone, which are later released by the pituitary gland.

THE PITUITARY GLAND, THE "ORCHESTRA CONDUCTOR" OF THE ENDOCRINE SYSTEM

The pituitary gland is closely related to the hypothalamus and is under the influence of its stimulating or inhibiting secretions. The pituitary gland **orchestrates** the activity in the endocrine system through its hormones, which act directly upon organic tissues or other endocrine glands. Actually, it **produces** seven hormones that regulate such diverse and fundamental things as body growth or that control the activity of the thyroid, adrenal cortex, and gonads. When needed, it **stores** and **releases** two hormones made by the hypothalamus: **antidiuretic hormone** and **oxytocin**.

> The activity of the hypothalamus and the pituitary gland are so closely related that they are usually referred to as the "hypothalamic-pituitary axis."

THE PINEAL GLAND, A MYSTERY

The pineal gland is a small structure, located in the brain, whose activity in human beings is not known with certainty. Its only function seems to be the secretion of **melatonin**, a hormone whose level in the blood fluctuates in a 24-hour cycle and reaches a maximum value during the night. It is possible, then, that the pineal gland is involved in **synchronizing the circadian rhythm** that different body functions have; but, this is still a mystery.

HORMONES OF THE PITUITARY GLAND

Name	Abbrev.	Target organ	Function
Melanocyte stimulating hormone	MSH	Skin	It stimulates melanocytes, the cells producing pigment, which gives the skin its color
Antidiuretic hormone	ADH	Kidneys	It causes water retention in the kidneys and is involved in the regulation of the blood pressure
Hydrocortisone, Somatropin hormone, Growth hormone	HC, STH, GH	Whole body	It stimulates the growth of bones, muscles, and all the organs in the body during childhood and puberty
Thyroid hormone	TSH	Thyroid	It stimulates the activity of the thyroid gland
Oxytocin		Uterus	It causes the contractions of the uterus during delivery
Adrenocorticotropic hormone	ACTH	Adrenal glands	They stimulate the production of corticosteroids in the adrenal glands
Prolactine	PRL	Breasts	It causes milk secretion after the delivery
Gonadotrophins Follicular stimulating hormone, Luteinizing hormone, Interstitial cell stimulating hormone	FSH, LH, ICSH	Gonads (ovaries and testes)	They regulate the sperm and egg maturation, and the production of sexual hormones

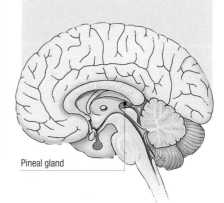

Pineal gland

THE ANTIDIURETIC HORMONE

The activity of the antidiuretic hormone, produced in the hypothalamus and released by the pituitary gland takes place in the kidneys: it controls the **reabsorption of water** in the renal tubules after filtering the blood in the glomerulus. For that reason, it tends to **reduce diuresis**, that is, the amount of excreted urine produced by the kidneys. When the secretion of this hormone fails, the affected person urinates much more than normal, and, if the loss is not replenished through drinking fluids, the person runs the risk of suffering a critical episode of **dehydration**. This hormone also causes **an increase in the volume of circulating blood** and **an increase in the blood pressure**, which explains the other name it receives: **vasopressin**. Various factors influence the production of this hormone, especially the concentration of solutes in the blood. If the concentration of solutes is very high, antidiuretic hormone is released to decrease the elimination of water in the kidneys, causing a greater dilution of the blood.

 Alcohol inhibits the production of antidiuretic hormone: that explains why after drinking an excessive amount of alcoholic drinks there is a large amount of urination.

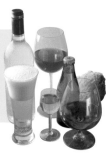

ACTION OF ANTIDIURETIC HORMONE

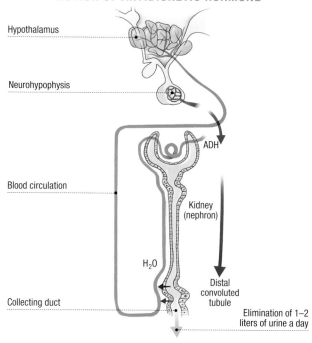

Hypothalamus

Neurohypophysis

ADH

Blood circulation

Kidney (nephron)

H_2O

Distal convoluted tubule

Collecting duct

Elimination of 1–2 liters of urine a day

REGULATION OF THE SECRETION OF ANTIDIURETIC HORMONE

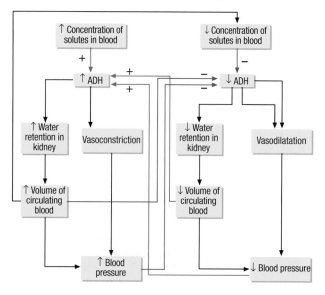

↑ Concentration of solutes in blood

↓ Concentration of solutes in blood

+

−

↑ ADH

↓ ADH

+

+

−

−

↑ Water retention in kidney

Vasoconstriction

↓ Water retention in kidney

Vasodilatation

↑ Volume of circulating blood

↓ Volume of circulating blood

↑ Blood pressure

↓ Blood pressure

THYROID FUNCTION

The function of the thyroid gland is of the utmost importance, because it produces hormones that stimulate cellular combustion, thereby activating **metabolism** and **heat production**. During childhood, the thyroid hormones definitively influence the **maturation of the nervous system** and **body growth**, conditioning **physical** and **mental development**. The two main thyroid hormones characterized by containing **iodine** are **thyroxin (T4)** and **triiodothyronine (T3)**. These hormones have a similar action: they cause, in all organic tissues, an increase in the metabolic reactions.

ARTIFICIAL HORMONES

Today it is possible to make different hormones for the **treatment** of many conditions and especially to give them when, for various reasons, there is a **production deficiency**. Some hormones can be obtained through **chemical synthesis** in the laboratory, whereas others are obtained through techniques of **genetic engineering**. That is the case of the growth hormone (GH), used to fight the deficiency in production responsible for the disorder known as pituitary dwarfism. It is now possible to obtain GH by using methods of biotechnology and in sufficient amounts to guarantee the treatment of all affected children.

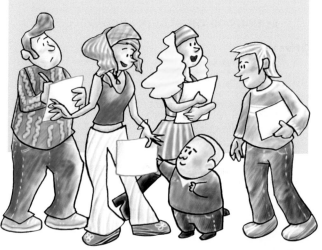

A deficiency in the production of growth hormone during childhood or puberty can give rise to a disorder called pituitary dwarfism: a defect of body development in which the person has a shorter height than normal. An excessive production of the hormone during that period causes a disorder known as gigantism, in which the person is taller than normal.

Introduction

A Perfect Machine

Skin

Digestive System

Nutrition

Respiratory System

Circulatory System and Blood

Nervous System

Musculoskeletal System

Urinary System

Endocrine System

Immune System

The Senses

Genetics

Reproductive System

Human Development

Index

REGULATION MECHANISM OF THE THYROID

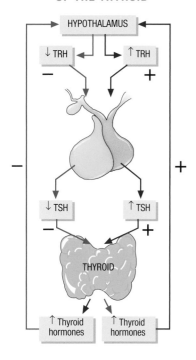

REGULATION OF THYROID ACTIVITY

Thyroid activity is controlled by the hypothalamic pituitary axis, because the gland responds to the stimulus of **thyrotropin (TSH)**, produced by the pituitary gland, whose production depends on the **thyrotropin-releasing factor (TRH)**, produced by the hypothalamus. The production of thyroid hormones is based on a **negative feedback mechanism**, blood concentration constituting the main condition for the hypothalamus and for pituitary activity. When the blood levels of thyroid hormones are high, the hypothalamus detects this and secretes less TRH, stopping the stimulation of the pituitary gland for the production of TSH. The production of thyrotropin decreases, the thyroid is less stimulated, and its hormonal production decreases. When the levels of thyroid hormone decrease too much, the hypothalamus increases the secretion of TRH, which acts upon the pituitary gland and causes an increase in the release of TSH. Then, thyrotropin production increases and this stimulates the thyroid activity.

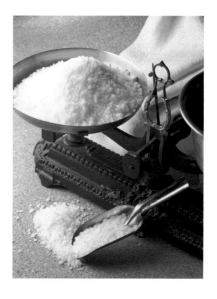

THYROID ACTIVITY

Under the stimulus of thyrotropin, the cells of the thyroid take **iodine (I)** from the blood, and they also synthesize a protein called **thyroglobulin**. In the center of the cell, iodine joins the thyroglobuline molecules, causing the formation of two products: **monoiodthyronine**, which has one atom of iodine, and **diiodothyronine**, which has two atoms of iodine. Another union of these products causes the formation of T3, which has three atoms of iodine, or T4, which has four. Once produced, the hormones are stored in the thyroid until they are released in the bloodstream, if needed, and are transported by the blood throughout the body to act upon the different tissues.

IMPORTANCE OF IODINE

Iodine is an essential micronutrient for the physical and intellectual development of people throughout life and especially during gestation and childhood. A diet deficient in iodine causes a deficiency of thyroid hormone, thereby causing a deficiency in brain growth and in the formation of the nervous system. Often, this results in a child with an incapacity for life. To guarantee enough iodine intake, it is now added to salt used for human and animal consumption. This is known as **universal salt iodization**.

ACTIONS OF THE PARATHYROID HORMONE

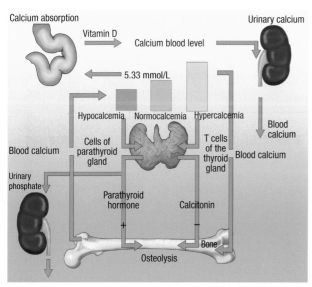

ROLE OF PARATHYROID GLANDS

The parathyroid glands are four tiny glands that produce **parathyroid hormone**, or **parathormone**, a substance that, with **calcitonin**, produced by the thyroid gland, and vitamin D, is involved in the regulation of the blood calcium level. Parathyroid hormone tends to **increase the calcium blood levels**; to do this, it acts on three different levels: on the bones, on the kidneys, and in the digestive tube. In the bones, it stimulates the activity of osteoclasts and therefore promotes the destruction of bone tissue. With that, the bones release into the blood part of their stored calcium. In the kidneys, it acts upon the renal tubules and increases the **reabsorption of calcium** filtered in the glomerulus, causing a **decrease in the elimination through urine** of this mineral, whose levels go up in the blood. In the digestive tube, it increases the intestinal absorption of calcium contained in food by means of activation of vitamin D at the kidney level. **Calcitonin** has the opposite effect; therefore, its action tends to decrease the blood levels of calcium: it inhibits bone destruction and decreases the renal reabsorption of calcium, causing an increase in the elimination through urine of the mineral.

ADRENAL GLANDS

The adrenal glands, or suprarenal glands because they are located on top of the kidneys, are made up of two completely different parts with different functions: the cortex, the largest part, and the medulla, which is in the center. The **adrenal cortex**, controlled by the hypothalamic-pituitary axis, produces hormones known as **corticosteroids**. There are different types of corticosteroids involved in the metabolism of nutrients, in the regulation of blood pressure, and in the development of secondary sexual characters. The **adrenal medulla** is under the control of the autonomic nervous system and produces hormones that act upon the whole body to achieve a better adaptation to stressful situations.

To fight inflammation and to treat allergic conditions, doctors usually prescribe corticoids, a medicine with very similar actions to those of the hormones produced by the adrenal cortex.

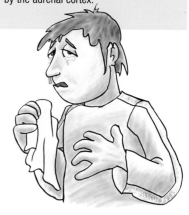

CIRCADIAN CYCLE

Adrenal cortex activity is regulated by both the hypothalamus and by the pituitary gland. The former produces the **corticotropin-releasing factor (CRF)**, which acts upon the latter, stimulating the production of **adreno-corticotropin**, a hormone that travels in the blood, reaching the adrenal glands and promoting the production of glucocorticoids and androgens. The secretion of all these substances is subject to a particular daily rhythm, the **circadian cycle**, in which increases and decreases related to sleeping and waking periods are observed. Basically, the blood levels of these hormones, which favor the availability of energy, are higher during the first hours of the morning, preparing the body for greater activity, whereas the levels go down during the night, when the body rests.

ROLE OF THE ADRENAL CORTEX

The adrenal cortex produces several hormones with a similar chemical structure. They belong to the **steroids** group but have different functions. One group of these hormones corresponds to **mineralocorticoids**, whose main component is aldosterone. These hormones are involved in the regulation of the balance of fluids and salts, especially sodium and potassium. They act on the kidneys and adapt water and salt losses through urine to body needs. Another group is made up of **glucocorticoids**, whose main component is the hormone called cortisol or hydrocortisone. Glucocorticoids regulate the metabolism of energetic nutrients and have a powerful anti-inflammatory action and immunodepressors, because they inhibit cellular immunity. A third group is made up of **androgens**, hormones promoting the development of male sexual characters and muscle tissue growth, the most important being dehydroepiandrosterone.

The hormones from the adrenal cortex are of great physiological importance; an animal cannot survive for long if an adrenal gland is removed.

ACTIVITY OF THE ADENAL CORTEX

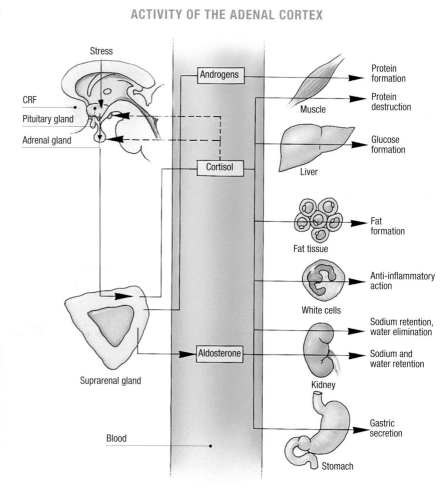

Stress

CRF

Pituitary gland

Adrenal gland

Androgens

Cortisol

Muscle — Protein formation / Protein destruction

Liver — Glucose formation

Fat tissue — Fat formation

White cells — Anti-inflammatory action

Aldosterone

Kidney — Sodium retention, water elimination / Sodium and water retention

Stomach — Gastric secretion

Suprarenal gland

Blood

ALDOSTERONE AND BLOOD PRESSURE

Aldosterone, produced by the adrenal cortex, takes part in **mineral** and **fluid balance** in the body. Its function takes place in the kidneys, where it increases sodium reabsorption and elimination of potassium through urine. These actions result in an increase of **liquid retention** in the body and therefore in an **increase in blood pressure**. Under normal conditions, aldosterone production depends on a delicate regulating mechanism. If there is a decrease in blood pressure, the kidneys secrete **renin**, a hormone that activates **angiotensin**, a substance made by the liver and present in the plasma. Angiotensin acts upon the adrenal cortex and stimulates the production and release of aldosterone.

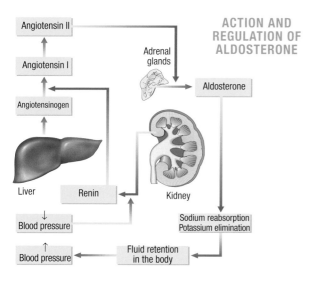

ACTION AND REGULATION OF ALDOSTERONE

Angiotensin II
Angiotensin I
Angiotensinogen
Adrenal glands
Aldosterone
Liver
Renin
Kidney
↓ Blood pressure
Sodium reabsorption Potassium elimination
↑ Blood pressure
Fluid retention in the body

REGULATION OF GLYCEMIA

The control of **blood glucose concentration** is very important, especially because it is the only substance that the nervous system can use directly as a **fuel** to obtain energy. The pancreas actively participates in this mechanism by means of its two hormones. When glycemia goes up, the pancreas releases insulin, whereas when glycemia levels are down, the secretion of insulin is reduced drastically. The objective of this regulating mechanism is to prevent glycemia from reaching certain ranges, because it is harmful if it goes up or down too much.

MECHANISMS OF GLYCEMIA REGULATION

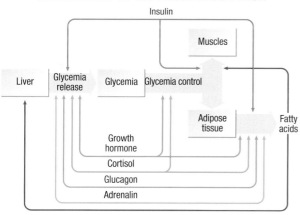

Insulin
Muscles
Liver
Glycemia release
Glycemia
Glycemia control
Adipose tissue
Fatty acids
Growth hormone
Cortisol
Glucagon
Adrenalin

FUNCTION OF THE ADRENAL MEDULLA

The adrenal medulla is made up of nerve tissue and produces two hormones that are part of a group known as **catecholamines**: **epinephrine** (adrenaline) and **norepinephrine** (noradrenline). These hormones are **neurotransmitters** released into the blood stream, when the body needs to face an intense physical activity or a difficult situation. They are usually referred to as "stress hormones," because they enter the blood circulation when there is a situation of danger. Under normal conditions, the adrenaline and noradrenline blood levels are low, but when needed, the levels go up quickly, and they are even able to increase in a matter of seconds. Catecholamines are secreted under the stimuli of the **sympathetic autonomic nervous system** and act upon a variety of organs and tissues in different ways: increasing the blood pressure, the heart rate, the blood flow in the skeletal muscles, the diameter of bronchi, the size of pupils, while decreasing the blood flow in the skin and the digestive abdominal organs.

ACTIONS OF INSULINE AND GLUCAGON

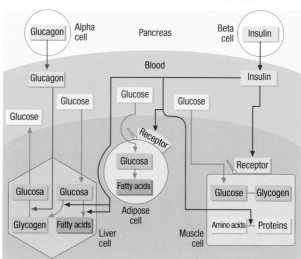

Glucagon — Alpha cell — Pancreas — Beta cell — Insulin
Glucagon
Blood
Insulin
Glucose
Glucose
Glucose
Receptor
Glucose
Glucosa
Receptor
Glucose — Glycogen
Glucosa — Glucosa
Fatty acids
Glycogen — Fatty acids — Adipose cell
Liver cell
Muscle cell
Amino acids — Proteins

THE ENDOCRINE PANCREAS

The pancreas, besides producing and releasing into the small intestine a secretion high in enzymes, thereby performing a fundamental role in the digestive process, also acts as an **endocrine gland**, because it produces two hormones that participate in the metabolism of carbohydrates and that **regulate blood glucose levels**. One of these, **insulin**, increases the passage of glucose from the blood to the inside of the cells, where it is used as a nutrient and as the main source of energy. The insulin action has a **hypoglycemic effect**, because it causes a decrease in the concentration of blood glucose. The other pancreatic hormone is **glucagon**, which has the opposite action from that of insulin and therefore has an **hyperglycemic effect**, because it promotes the breaking down of glycogen stored in the cells and the passage of glucose to the blood.

If the pancreas does not produce enough insulin, the result is an illness called diabetes. People with diabetes must give themselves daily insulin injections.

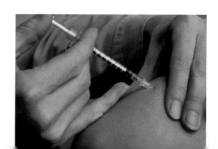

THE IMMUNE SYSTEM

The immune system corresponds to the **defense system** of the body, because it has several mechanisms, mainly carried out by **white cells**, to protect us from possible attacks of **dangerous foreign** **elements** coming from the outside world, especially **germs** and **microbes**, which are always present in our environment.

LYMPHOID ORGANS

Lymphoid organs are structures where the various white cells responsible for immune actions are produced, mature, and acquire their distinctive features. The main organ is **bone marrow**, located inside the different bones of the body. It is constantly making white cells that enter the blood and, later, some of them enter body tissues. Another important organ is the **thymus**, which has an essential function. During the fetal life, many lymphocytes mature and "learn" to **recognize the elements** **belonging** to the body and so they are able to detect any **foreign element** that enters the body. **Lymph nodes** are also very important and are placed along the path of the lymph vessels, where some white cells reproduce. Finally, the **spleen** is also considered a lymphoid organ, because some white cells reproduce these, and these later enter the bloodstream.

ORGANS OF THE IMMUNE SYSTEM

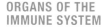

Thymus

An organ where white cells of the type lymphocyte T mature and become able to perform their specific function during gestation and childhood

Lymph nodes

Small lymphoid organs spread throughout the body and placed along passages of lymph vessels; they work as a filter for germs and impurities

Spleen

The organ where some types of white cells reproduce, acting as a filter for germs and impurities in blood

Peyer's patches (Illiac nodes)

Lymphoid groups located in the intestine

Bone marrow

A tissue that makes most of the white cells, the main component of the immune system

MODERATE EXERCISE

Excessive exercise can be harmful for the immune system, weakening our defenses. However, the opposite happens when you do moderate exercise, which boosts the immune system.

LYMPH NODES: NATURAL FILTERS

The numerous lymph nodes spread throughout the body are of great importance for the defense of our bodies. They house a large number of white cells in charge of **detecting** and **neutralizing**, or **destroying**, germs or impurities transported by lymph vessels that drain the body tissues. Each node is made up of a **capsule** of connective tissue from which some trabeculi arise, dividing the nodule into several portions containing lymphoid follicles full of white cells. **Afferent lymph vessels** reach the node transporting the lymph picked up in the tissues. The lymph is then filtered and freed of harmful elements, or potentially dangerous ones, and comes out through the **efferent lymph vessels** and continues its path toward the circulatory system. Because the lymph nodes are located in strategic places in the body, their action prevents the spread of harmful agents.

STRUCTURE OF A LYMPH NODE

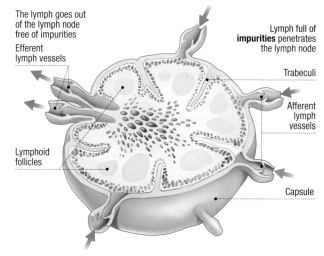

The lymph goes out of the lymph node free of impurities

Efferent lymph vessels

Lymphoid follicles

Lymph full of **impurities** penetrates the lymph node

Trabeculi

Afferent lymph vessels

Capsule

NONSPECIFIC IMMUNITY: INNATE DEFENSE

FUNCTION OF WHITE CELLS

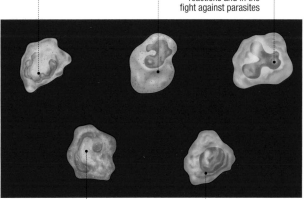

Neutrophil
Acts as a phagocyte

Basophil
Takes part in allergic reactions

Eosinophil
Takes part in allergic reactions and in the fight against parasites

Lymphocyte
Takes part in immune responses

Monocyte
Acts as a phagocyte

The body has a series of resources to protect itself in a nonspecific way against the attack of potentially pathogenic germs. First, there are **protective barriers**, such as the skin, which prevents germs from entering, and several fluids, such as nasal mucous, saliva, or tears, containing enzymes that are able to destroy many microbes. If germs manage to penetrate these defense lines, they will face the action of phagocytes, white cells traveling throughout the body that eat and digest all foreign particles they encounter. Germs will also have to face the group of plasma proteins, which constitute a supplementary system, able to attack the walls of germs and destroy them or to facilitate the action of white cells.

PHAGOCYTOSIS MECHANISM

Nucleus

Phagocyte

Bacteria

Waste products eliminated

Waste products

Phagocytes modify their shape and engulf the microbe

A vacuum space forms that traps the microbe

The enzymes that will digest the microbe are released in the vacuum space

The phagocyte goes back to normal

SPECIFIC IMMUNITY: ACQUIRED DEFENSE

If any microorganism manages to go through the first defense mechanisms, a **specific immune reaction** starts with the purpose of protecting the body exclusively against each attacking agent. The defensive response in charge of the white cells is based on recognition of the foreign agent's structural elements, called **antigens**, and on activating a series of **cell** and **humoral mechanisms** to destroy or neutralize the attacker. **Cellular immune response** corresponds to **lymphocyte T cells**. There are different varieties of T cells; some detect the germ and secrete chemical substances that generate a warning signal in

the area, whereas others behave as "**killer cells**" that attack the microbe, destroying it. **Humoral immune response** corresponds to **lymphocyte B cells**, which when faced with a warning sign, multiply and turn into **plasma cells** in charge of producing **antibodies**; that is to say, **gamma globulin** that joins the attacking germ's antigens and facilitates the attack of immune cells present in the area. Some of these lymphocytes "**remember**" the attacking germ to act sooner and more efficiently should the germ enter the body again, thus generating a state of **immunization**.

MECHANISMS OF SPECIFIC IMMUNITY

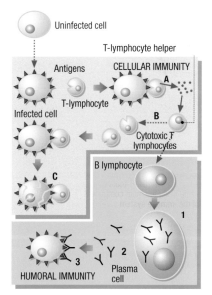

Uninfected cell

T-lymphocyte helper

Antigens

CELLULAR IMMUNITY

T-lymphocyte

Infected cell

Cytotoxic T lymphocytes

B lymphocyte

Plasma cell

HUMORAL IMMUNITY

A. Lymphocyte T cells recognize the antigen and release chemical substances
B. Helper lymphocyte T cells capture the signal and as a response, they activate cytotoxic lymphocyte T cells and lymphocyte B cells
C. Cytotoxic lymphocyte T cells join the antigens and destroy the cell
1. Lymphocyte B cells are different in plasmatic cells
2. Plasma cells release antibodies
3. Antibodies join antigens and destroy or deactivate the infectious germ

VACCINATIONS

Vaccination is an ingenious prophylactic medical procedure that allows us to prevent infection from several infectious diseases. It is based on "tricking" the immune system: the germ responsible for a disease is injected, but deprived of its power; that is to say, it is deactivated in the laboratory. The defense system "believes" it is being attacked and so generates an immune response without having to suffer the illness.

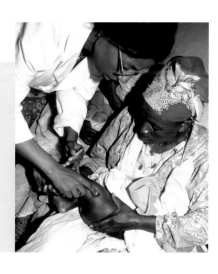

THE SENSES, WINDOWS TO THE WORLD

Our senses of sight, hearing, taste, smell, and touch have a fundamental function. They allow us to perceive several types of **stimuli** from outside, and they provide us with **information** about the environment and about what goes on around us, an essential factor for keeping us connected to the surrounding reality.

EYE COMPONENTS

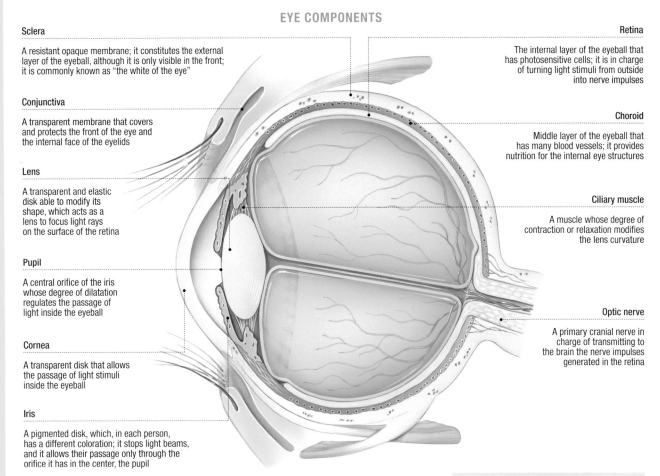

Sclera

A resistant opaque membrane; it constitutes the external layer of the eyeball, although it is only visible in the front; it is commonly known as "the white of the eye"

Conjunctiva

A transparent membrane that covers and protects the front of the eye and the internal face of the eyelids

Lens

A transparent and elastic disk able to modify its shape, which acts as a lens to focus light rays on the surface of the retina

Pupil

A central orifice of the iris whose degree of dilatation regulates the passage of light inside the eyeball

Cornea

A transparent disk that allows the passage of light stimuli inside the eyeball

Iris

A pigmented disk, which, in each person, has a different coloration; it stops light beams, and it allows their passage only through the orifice it has in the center, the pupil

Retina

The internal layer of the eyeball that has photosensitive cells; it is in charge of turning light stimuli from outside into nerve impulses

Choroid

Middle layer of the eyeball that has many blood vessels; it provides nutrition for the internal eye structures

Ciliary muscle

A muscle whose degree of contraction or relaxation modifies the lens curvature

Optic nerve

A primary cranial nerve in charge of transmitting to the brain the nerve impulses generated in the retina

FUNCTION OF THE EYE

The eye, also called the **eyeball**, is the organ of sight. It is a complex anatomical structure responsible for receiving **light stimuli** coming from outside and turning these stimuli into **nerve impulses** that are transmitted by the optic nerve to the brain to be decoded and **interpreted as images**. Its functioning can be compared with a photographic camera or, better yet, to a video camera, because it allows us to have a continuous visual representation of the world around us. If we develop the simile of the photographic camera, the **sclera**, which is the external cover, corresponds to the chassis. The **iris** acts as a diaphragm, because the contraction and dilation of the pupil regulates the passage of light to the inside. The **lens** works as a lens, because it focuses the light beams onto the **retina**, which is sensitive to light stimuli, like photographic film.

LENS ACCOMODATION MECHANISM

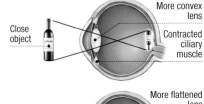

Close object — More convex lens — Contracted ciliary muscle

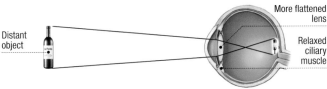

Distant object — More flattened lens — Relaxed ciliary muscle

FOCUSING ON OBJECTS

To **see** objects **clearly**, it is necessary that their image form on the retina; otherwise they would look blurry. The **optical system** has elements, such as the cornea and the lens, that are adapted for seeing in the distance. The lens, a biconvex disk, has a relatively flattened shape so that light beams coming from far objects are **focused onto the retina**, and a **clear image** can be seen. Short sight vision is different: if no changes were made, the image of objects located a few feet away would look blurry. This does not happen, because the eye has a mechanism called **accommodation**. When we look at a nearby object, the ciliary muscle contracts and the lens changes its shape so that light beams bend as needed to be focused perfectly on the retina.

Introduction

A Perfect
Machine

Skin

Digestive
System

Nutrition

Respiratory
System

Circulatory
System and
Blood

Nervous
System

Musculoskeletal
System

Urinary
System

Endocrine
System

Immune
System

The Senses

Genetics

Reproductive
System

Human
Development

Index

PROJECTION OF IMAGES IN THE RETINA

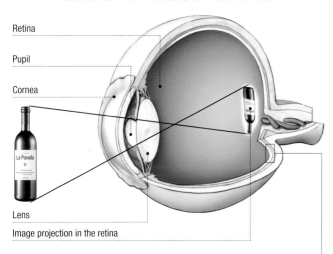

Retina

Pupil

Cornea

Lens

Image projection in the retina

FUNCTION OF RETINA

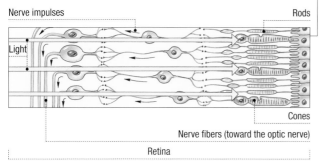

Nerve impulses

Rods

Light

Cones

Nerve fibers (toward the optic nerve)

Retina

Approximately 5% of males and 1% of females cannot tell all colors apart clearly and above all cannot perceive red, green, or blue. They suffer a hereditary disorder called daltonism (color blindness).

VISUAL PATHWAYS

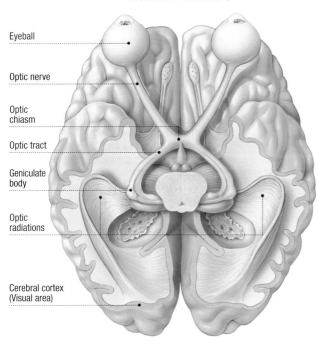

Eyeball

Optic nerve

Optic chiasm

Optic tract

Geniculate body

Optic radiations

Cerebral cortex (Visual area)

IMAGE PERCEPTION

Light beams given off by an external object, after being focused by the lens, continue their path and **intersect** at a focal point before reaching the surface of the retina, where an **inverted image** is formed. This inverted image is later decoded and interpreted by the brain in its original position. In the retina, there are two types of **photoreceptors** that turn those light stimuli into **nerve impulses**. **Cones** react in a lighted environment and are sensitive to colors. **Rods** react in environments with little light and provide black and white vision. Nerve impulses generated in photoreceptors are transmitted to the cells, whose extensions constitute the optic nerve, in charge of driving them to the brain.

TEST: CAN I TELL COLORS APART?

The photoreceptors of the retina are sensitive to colors. There are three types of cones. Some cones are stimulated by red, others by green, and still others by blue. But simultaneous stimulation of the three types allows us to distinguish a wide variety of **chromatic shades**. Here are some pictures with dots of different colors; in the middle there are some dots in one color that form letters or numbers used to check if chromatic vision works perfectly and if all shades can be perceived, without confusing them. Look at these pictures closely, and, if your chromatic vision is good, you will be able to see from left to right and downward the following symbols: 182, 13, F4, 69.

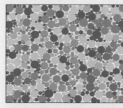
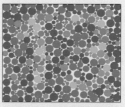
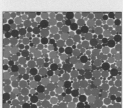
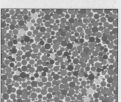

PATH OF VISUAL STIMULI

Nerve impulses generated in cones and rods come out from the eye through the optic nerve and follow a long path until they reach the brain. The two optic nerves, each coming from an eye, pass by the inferior part of the brain and join at the **optic chiasm**, where a part of the nerve fibers from both intertwine. The **optic tracts** start there, carrying the information to the **external geniculate bodies** of the optic thalamus, where some new neurons take over and transmit the impulses through **optic radiations** to the cerebral cortex of the occipital lobe, seat of the **visual area**. It is in this area where nerve impulses from the eyes turn into visual sensations; perceptions turn into consciousness by mechanisms not yet fully known.

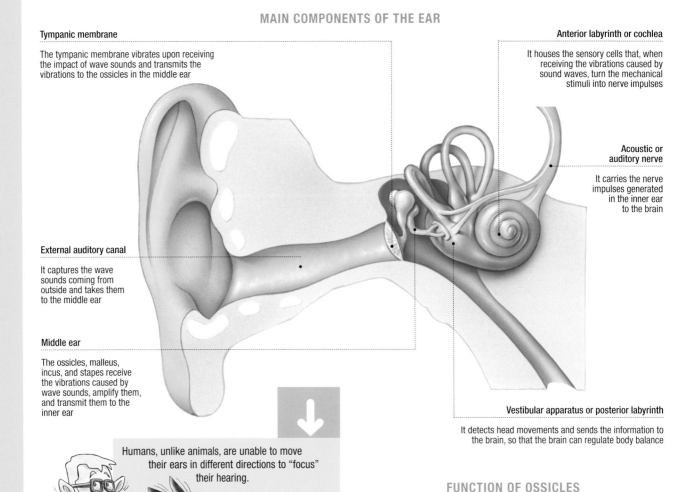

Tympanic membrane

The tympanic membrane vibrates upon receiving the impact of wave sounds and transmits the vibrations to the ossicles in the middle ear

Anterior labyrinth or cochlea

It houses the sensory cells that, when receiving the vibrations caused by sound waves, turn the mechanical stimuli into nerve impulses

Acoustic or auditory nerve

It carries the nerve impulses generated in the inner ear to the brain

External auditory canal

It captures the wave sounds coming from outside and takes them to the middle ear

Middle ear

The ossicles, malleus, incus, and stapes receive the vibrations caused by wave sounds, amplify them, and transmit them to the inner ear

Vestibular apparatus or posterior labyrinth

It detects head movements and sends the information to the brain, so that the brain can regulate body balance

Humans, unlike animals, are able to move their ears in different directions to "focus" their hearing.

FUNCTION AND STRUCTURE OF THE EAR

The ear has two functions. On the one hand, it is responsible for **hearing**, a very important sense for perceiving what goes on around us, and a fundamental tool for **communication**, because **spoken language** is the main means of communication among humans. On the other hand, the ear takes part in **body balance**, because it provides the brain with information about head positions and movements, so that our muscles keep adapting to momentary changes, and we are able to keep our balance when standing or walking. The organ is very complex and is divided into three portions, each having a different role. The **external ear**, formed by the outer ear and the external auditory canal, only takes part in hearing. The same is true of the **middle ear**, which is separated from the external ear by the tympanic membrane and which contains a chain of ossicles: malleus, incus, and stape. However, **the inner ear**, also called the labyrinth, is made up of two portions with different functions: the **anterior labyrinth**, or **cochlea**, where the organ of Corti, responsible for hearing, is located, and the **posterior labyrinth**, or **vestibular apparatus**, which takes part in maintaining balance.

FUNCTION OF OSSICLES IN THE MIDDLE EAR

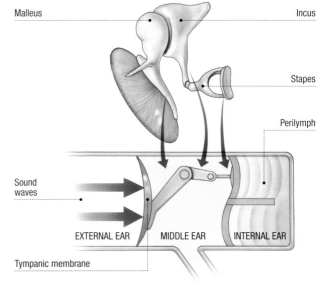

Malleus

Incus

Stapes

Perilymph

Sound waves

Tympanic membrane

EXTERNAL EAR   MIDDLE EAR   INTERNAL EAR

When vibrating, the tympanic membrane moves the chain of ossicles of the middle ear. Each vibration causes the movement of the malleus, the malleus moves the incus, and the latter moves the stapes. The base of the stapes impacts with the oval window, and the sound concentrates and intensifies on its path through the ossicles to compensate for the loss of energy suffered by sound waves when passing from an air medium to a liquid one. Due to this mechanism, the weakest sounds can be perceived.

Introduction

A Perfect
Machine

Skin

Digestive
System

Nutrition

Respiratory
System

Circulatory
System and
Blood

Nervous
System

Musculoskeletal
System

Urinary
System

Endocrine
System

Immune
System

The Senses

Genetics

Reproductive
System

Human
Development

Index

PHYSIOLOGY OF HEARING

Hearing is based on transforming **sound waves**, corresponding to **vibrations of air molecules** spreading from the point where a sound is produced into nerve impulses that the brain decodes. The sound waves are picked up by the ear and are transmitted through the **external auditory canal** to the **tympanic membrane**, a membrane that separates the outer ear from the middle ear. The vibrations are transmitted to the **ossicles**, in the middle ear, and then vibrate on the **oval window**, to allow their passage to the inner ear, which is full of liquid. When the oval window vibrates, a movement of the perilymph results and produces a wave that travels along the cochlea, first along the **vestibular duct**, and then along the **tympanic duct** until it fades in the **round window**. On its path, the perilymph movement causes the **basilar membrane**, the base of the **cochlea**, to vibrate. The **organ of Corti**, a basic element in hearing, is located in the cochlea. When sensory cells move because of vibrations, the small cilia on their upper surfaces impinge on the tectorial membrane, generating metabolic changes that turn the mechanical impulses into nerve impulses that are transmitted to the fibers of the **cochlear nerve** and that reach the brain through the **auditory nerve**, where sound perception is made conscious.

HEARING MECHANISM

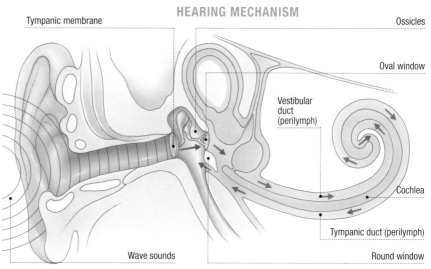

Tympanic membrane
Ossicles
Oval window
Vestibular duct (perilymph)
Cochlea
Tympanic duct (perilymph)
Wave sounds
Round window

HEARING MECHANISM IN THE INNER EAR

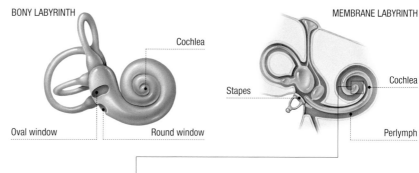

BONY LABYRINTH

Cochlea

Oval window
Round window

MEMBRANE LABYRINTH

Stapes
Cochlea
Perilymph

RANGE OF SOUND FREQUENCIES HEARD BY HUMANS AND OTHER ANIMALS

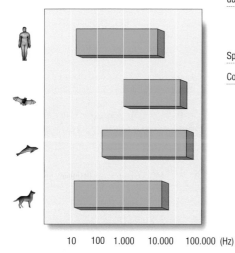

10   100   1.000   10.000   100.000 (Hz)

The human ear can only capture wave sounds in a frequency range between 16 and 20,000 hertz or vibrations per second, whereas some animals can perceive infrasound of lower frequencies, and others can perceive ultrasounds of higher frequencies, inaudible to humans.

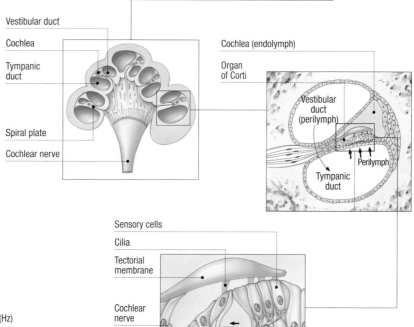

Vestibular duct
Cochlea
Tympanic duct

Spiral plate
Cochlear nerve

Cochlea (endolymph)
Organ of Corti

Vestibular duct (perilymph)
Perilymph
Tympanic duct

Sensory cells
Cilia
Tectorial membrane
Cochlear nerve
Nerve impulses
Perilymph
Basilar membrane

TASTE

Taste is the sense that allows us to know special characteristics of everything we drink and eat. Many animals are guided by this sense to **select their food**. Human beings are not as reliable; there are some very nutritious meals we do not like; there are others that, from a nutritional point of view, have less value yet seem delicious to us. The taste of food is important when **making use of nutrients**, because when we like the food we eat, the production of digestive juices as a reflex increases. Taste receptors, **taste buds**, are located on the **tongue** and, in lesser numbers, on the palate and the throat. There are different types of taste buds, but they all have **corpuscles** or **taste buds** formed by a set of **sensory cells** located around a central cavity, the **taste pore**. When food enters the mouth, it mixes with saliva, and the soluble substances it contains enter the taste pores, causing a stimulus in the sensory cells. **Taste stimuli** go out through the nerve endings and travel through various nerves in the mouth to the **medulla**. From there, they go through other specific nerve pathways to the **thalamus**, and, in a third stage, they reach the **taste area**, located in the parietal lobe of the **cerebral cortex**, where they are decoded and sensations are made conscious.

TASTE BUDS ON THE TONGUE

Approximately 10,000 taste buds are spread all over the tongue's surface

Filiform papillae

Calciform papillae

Fungiform papillae

Calciform papillae

Fungiform papillae

Filiform papillae

Gustatory pore

Taste bud

Nerve endings

TASTE ZONES

Taste buds recognize **four basic taste** sensations that we all know very well: sweet, bitter, sour, and salty. The brain, when combining the different stimuli, is able to recognize many foods perfectly. All taste receptors on the tongue perceive the four basic tastes, but some react more intensely to some of the stimuli. This causes the existence of different areas where taste perception is more specialized. **Sweet** taste is perceived on the tip of the tongue, **bitter** taste on the back, **sour** taste on the edges, and **salty** taste is perceived on the front of the tongue, except on the tip.

TASTE PATHWAYS

Cerebral cortex

Thalamus

Facial and trigeminal nerves

Medulla oblongata

Vagus nerve

Glossopharangeal nerve

TASTE AREAS ON THE TONGUE

Bitter

Salty

Sour

Sweet

SMELL

Smell is the sense by which we perceive **odors**. This sense has different functions: it **takes part in digestion** because appetizing smells stimulate the production of gastric juices; it warns us about **dangerous gases** and plays an important role in love life, because it provides us with pleasant and unpleasant **sensations**. The receptors of this sense are in the **olfactory membrane**, a small area on the roof of the nostrils having a layer of cells specialized in the detection of smells. These cells are elongated and, on their free endings, have some minute **olfactory cilia** immersed in a mucous layer made by the glands on the nasal wall. **Air molecules** in the air we inhale, after dissolving in the mucous, attach to the reception areas of the cilia and generate nerve stimuli in cells. Olfactory cells have some thin nerve fibers that go through the roof of the nostrils and reach the **olfactory bulb**, from where the **olfactory nerve** carries the information to the olfactory centers of the **cerebral cortex**.

OLFACTORY MECHANISM

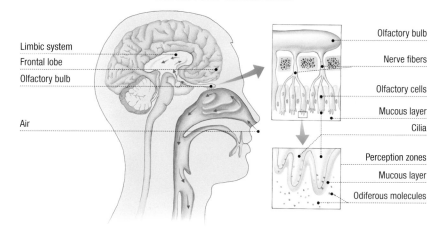

Limbic system
Frontal lobe
Olfactory bulb

Air

Olfactory bulb
Nerve fibers
Olfactory cells
Mucous layer
Cilia

Perception zones
Mucous layer
Odiferous molecules

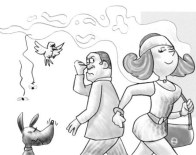

Olfactory cells "wear out" if exposed for a long time to the same substance. This explains why we get used to strong odors, pleasant (perfume) or disgusting (rotten smell) ones and after a while we stop smelling them.

TOUCH

Touch is a sense that provides us with valuable information about the world around us. It allows us to perceive **rubbing** and **pressure**, to identify the **shape** and **texture** of objects, to distinguish **variations in temperature**, and to notice external attacks when they cause **painful stimuli**. There are a multitude of combinations difficult to define but that we all know, such as itching or tickling. The touch organ is the **skin**, on whose surface thousands of receptors, which respond to various stimuli and which send information through the **sensory pathways** to the central

nervous system to be interpreted, are distributed. This function is performed by the **free endings of sensory nerves**, which reach the skin and perceive touch stimuli, but especially painful ones. Other special formations constitute **receptors specialized** in the perception of various stimuli. The **Vater-Pacini corpuscles** can detect the changes in pressure and the vibrations produced on the skin and its stretching; **Meissner corpuscles** respond to touch stimuli; **Krause corpuscles** are sensitive to cold; **Ruffini corpuscles** are sensitive to heat.

LEARNING TO PALPATE

The ability to recognize touch stimuli varies considerably in the different parts of the body, since perception is finer in areas where the skin is thinner and has many receptors. For example, on the fingertips, it is possible to distinguish even weak stimuli only one millimeter apart, while in some areas on the back two different stimuli applied at the same time even a couple of centimeters apart are perceived as one sensation. It is worth mentioning, however, that the ability to discriminate between touch stimuli can be widely developed with practice. That is the case in many professions: doctors are trained to appreciate minimal differences when palpating the body of a patient; for sculptors and craftsmen, touching is a basic tool, as it is for technicians handling small pieces of equipment.

TOUCH RECEPTORS ON THE SKIN

Meissner corpuscle

Krause corpuscle

Ruffini corpuscle

Vater-Pacini corpuscle

Free nerve endings

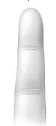

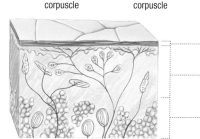
Epidermis

Dermis

Hypodermis

There is the Braille system for those who lack vision. The system consists of a series of raised dots that take the place of letters and that can be read by sliding the fingers over them.

GENETICS

Physical characteristics and the functioning of the body depend on the information stored in the **genes** inside the **DNA** that makes up the **chromosomes** present in the nucleus of cells. This constitutes an "instruction manual" that through **inheritance** passes traits to descendants and makes it possible to **continue the species** but, at the same time, determines that each individual has unique and unrepeatable features.

DNA, BASIC SUBSTANCE

DNA is short for **deoxyribonucleic acid**. It is formed by two long, parallel chains, coiled like a **double helix**, made up of sugar phosphate groups and **nitrogenous bases** of four kinds: adenine (A), guanine (G), thymine (T), and cytosine (C). Each chain is formed by a series of **nucleotides**, elements made up of one phosphate molecule, one deoxyribose molecule, and a nitrogenous base, linked to each other by a hydrogen bond. As a whole, the DNA double helix can be compared structurally with a spiral staircase. The link between the nitrogenous bases from both chains is not random, because it respects a strict rule. "A" only relates to "T," and "C" only relates to "G." Thus, the **base sequence** of a chain determines the sequence of another, a key factor for the replication of DNA when cellular division happens.

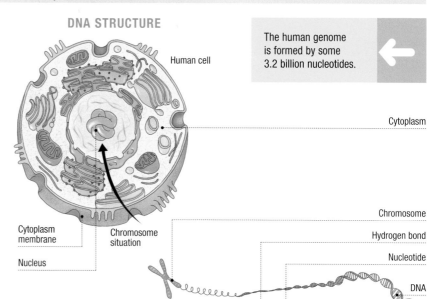

DNA STRUCTURE

Human cell

The human genome is formed by some 3.2 billion nucleotides.

Cytoplasm

Cytoplasm membrane

Chromosome situation

Nucleus

Chromosome

Hydrogen bond

Nucleotide

DNA

Nitrogenous Bases
Guanine
Adenine
Thymine
Cytosine

CHROMOSOMES

Inside the cellular nucleus, DNA forms a substance called **chromatin**. During the period in between cellular divisions, chromatin is scattered inside the nucleus, but when the moment of cellular division approaches, it condenses and constitutes some structures in the shape of rods, called **chromosomes**. Although there are chromosomes of different sizes, they all have a similar shape: a tiny rod with a constriction, the centromere, dividing into two arms, usually of unequal length. However, the image of the chromosomes that is usually seen corresponds to a stage of the process of cellular division in which the DNA has already replicated. Therefore, in that moment, two chromosomes can be observed, called **chromatids**, joined at the centromere: the shape of the set corresponds to an X, with two short arms and two long arms.

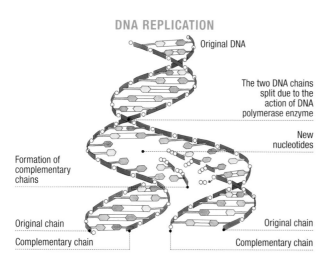

DNA REPLICATION

Original DNA

The two DNA chains split due to the action of DNA polymerase enzyme

New nucleotides

Formation of complementary chains

Original chain

Complementary chain

Original chain

Complementary chain

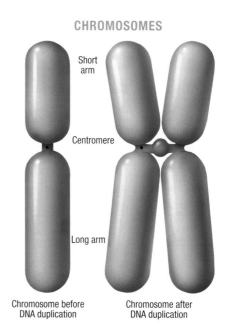

CHROMOSOMES

Short arm

Centromere

Long arm

Chromosome before DNA duplication

Chromosome after DNA duplication

CHROMOSOME SET

Organic cells 46 chromosomes

Organic cells 46 chromosomes

Ovum 23 chromosomes

Sperm 23 chromosomes

Fertilization

Egg cell 46 chromosomes

Organic cells 46 chromosomes

GENES

Genes are the **functional units** of the chromosomes, because each one corresponds to a specific portion of DNA and has a concrete role: **encoding** the necessary information for the synthesis of protein. In the sets of chromosomes, there are some 50,000 genes that encode structural body proteins or others with diverse functions, such as enzymes, hormones, etc. Each gene occupies a specific place in a certain chromosome, and, nowadays, its location is known with accuracy, so there is a "chromosome map," known as the **human genome**. In general terms, genes contain the instructions for the **production of proteins**, made up of a specific combination of **amino acids**. Although, there are thousands of different proteins, they are all formed by 20 different amino acids, and their combination is encoded in the genes. The mechanism that rules the **genetic code** is based on the sequence of nitrogenous bases of DNA fragments corresponding to the different genes. The four types of nitrogenous bases form a kind of **alphabet** whose reading is made in groups of three: each **triplet** encodes an amino acid; and the series of triplets read on and on, determines the composition of the polypeptide chain.

HUMAN CHROMOSOME SET

All the cells in the human body have **46 chromosomes**, except gametes, ova, and sperm, which only have half. Actually, there are **23 pairs of chromosome homologs** that are similar or equivalent. Out of these, 22 pairs are called **autosomes**, and both components in each pair are identical in all individuals. The remainder corresponds to **sexual chromosomes**, which are different in males and females. In females, the pair is made up of two **X chromosomes**, whereas in males, it is made up of an X chromosome and a **Y chromosome**. Because each gamete has 23 chromosomes, one of each pair, when the female one joins the male one in the

moment of fertilization, a cell with 23 pairs of chromosomes is formed. The division creates a new being.

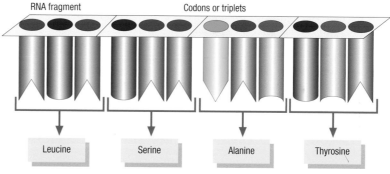

THE GENETIC CODE

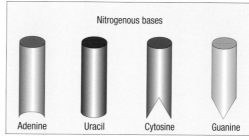

Nitrogenous bases

Adenine   Uracil   Cytosine   Guanine

RNA fragment

Codons or triplets

Leucine   Serine   Alanine   Thyrosine

Amino acid codes

Inheritance

Inheritance consists of the transmission of anatomical and physiological features from the biological parents to their descendants. The chromosome set of an individual corresponds to the sum of chromosomes from the ovum and sperm that join in fertilization, half contributed by the mother and the other half by the father. Therefore, each person has a gene that encodes certain data in each of the two chromosome homologs; but it is worth mentioning that there are genes that, although they have the same role, have variants called **alleles**. For

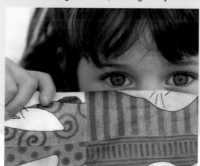

example, the gene that determines the eye color has variants responsible for the blue or brown coloration in the iris. Sometimes, the information contained in one allele dominates that in another: the first is **dominant**, whereas the second one is **recessive**.

THE REPRODUCTIVE SYSTEM

The reproductive system is made up of a set of organs, adapted to allow males and females to perform their sexual activity and especially to procreate.

COMPONENTS OF THE MALE REPRODUCTIVE SYSTEM

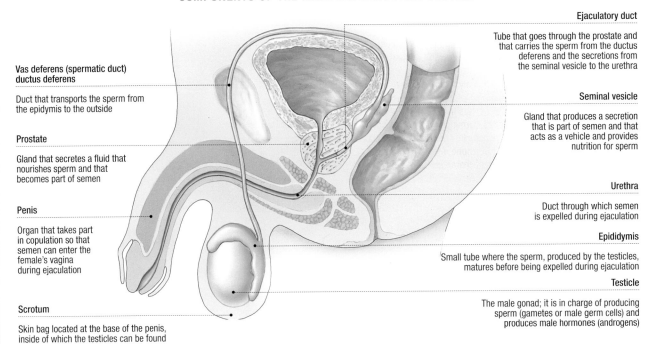

Vas deferens (spermatic duct) ductus deferens

Duct that transports the sperm from the epidymis to the outside

Prostate

Gland that secretes a fluid that nourishes sperm and that becomes part of semen

Penis

Organ that takes part in copulation so that semen can enter the female's vagina during ejaculation

Scrotum

Skin bag located at the base of the penis, inside of which the testicles can be found

Ejaculatory duct

Tube that goes through the prostate and that carries the sperm from the ductus deferens and the secretions from the seminal vesicle to the urethra

Seminal vesicle

Gland that produces a secretion that is part of semen and that acts as a vehicle and provides nutrition for sperm

Urethra

Duct through which semen is expelled during ejaculation

Epididymis

Small tube where the sperm, produced by the testicles, matures before being expelled during ejaculation

Testicle

The male gonad; it is in charge of producing sperm (gametes or male germ cells) and produces male hormones (androgens)

STRUCTURE OF SCROTUM

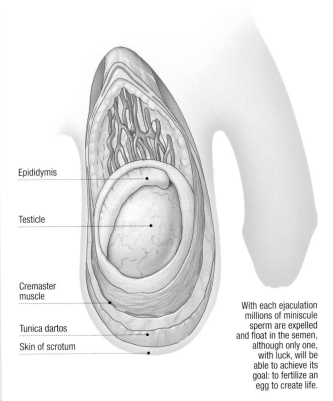

Epididymis

Testicle

Cremaster muscle

Tunica dartos

Skin of scrotum

With each ejaculation millions of miniscule sperm are expelled and float in the semen, although only one, with luck, will be able to achieve its goal: to fertilize an egg to create life.

FUNCTION OF THE SCROTUM

The scrotum has the very important function of keeping the testes **outside the abdominal cavity** and at a slightly lower temperature than the one inside the body. This is more appropriate for generating sperm. To carry out such an important job, the walls of the scrotum are made up of several layers. One of the layers, the most external one, is comprised of thin and **wrinkled skin**, with more or less deep grooves and under a muscular layer whose degree of contraction or relaxation modifies the depth of the skin grooves and the temperature at which the testes are exposed. When the temperature of the environment is high, the muscle relaxes and the grooves become less deep with a resulting **heat loss**. When the temperature is low, the muscle fibers contract and the skin grooves become deeper, decreasing the heat loss.

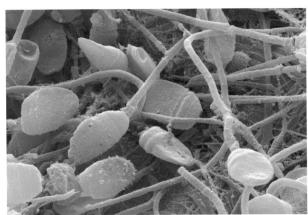

Introduction

A Perfect Machine

Skin

Digestive System

Nutrition

Respiratory System

Circulatory System and Blood

Nervous System

Musculoskeletal System

Urinary System

Endocrine System

Immune System

The Senses

Genetics

Reproductive System

Human Development

Index

FUNCTION OF TESTICLES

Testes have two functions: on the one hand, they are in charge of **producing sperm**, and, on the other hand, they have an **endocrine activity**. Both functions are regulated by pituitary gonadotrophins. Sperm production, or **spermatogenesis**, starts during puberty and takes place in the tiny seminiferous tubules, which have, since the embryonic stage, numerous **spermatogonia**, male germinal cells having 46 chromosomes. These cells reproduce and turn into **primary spermatocytes** under the influence of a hormone called FSH (follicle stimulating hormone). Then, they divide further, becoming **secondary spermatocytes**, which also have 46 chromosomes. These divide by a special mechanism, called **meiosis**, generating **spermatids**, with only 23 chromosomes: half with sexual chromosome X and the other half with sexual chromosome Y. Finally, the last stage of the process occurs in the epididymis, and the spermatids become spermatozoa, germinal mature cells having motility that start a long path to the outside. The testes also produce **testosterone**, the main **masculine hormone**, responsible for the development of secondary male sexual characteristics.

SPERMATOGENESIS

Spermatids

Sperm

22 chromosomes

22 chromosomes

+ X

+ Y

Secondary spermatocytes

44 chromosomes

+ X Y

Primary spermatocytes

Spermatogonia

Testes

Pituitary gland

FSH

Seminiferous tubules

ERECTION

Erection is the mechanism by which the penis, which is normally flaccid, **increases its size** and **consistency** in preparation for copulation. This mechanism is **involuntary**, is under the control of the parasympathetic autonomic nervous system, and is part of the male sexual response when there is an appropriate stimulus, either physical or psychological. In such a case, the arteries carrying blood to the penis dilate and this increases the blood flow going to the **erectile bodies** inside the penis, formed by trabecules that expand and fill with blood. At the same time this causes a compression in the veins in charge of draining blood from erectile bodies, which produces a stagnation of blood inside. As the erectile bodies fill, the penis goes from flaccidity to erection. It increases its size, especially in length, but also in thickness; it becomes rigid and it rises, pointing upward, creating the favorable conditions for sexual intercourse. After ejaculation, or if the sexual stimulus stops, the blood flow going to the penis decreases and the erectile bodies discharge their contents into the veins, and with that, the penis goes back to its flaccid state.

ACTION OF PITUITARY GONADOTROPHINS ON TESTES

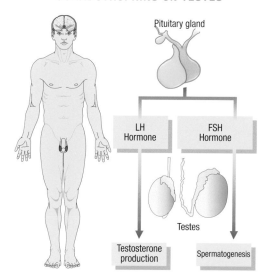

Pituitary gland

LH Hormone

FSH Hormone

Testes

Testosterone production

Spermatogenesis

ERECTION MECHANISM

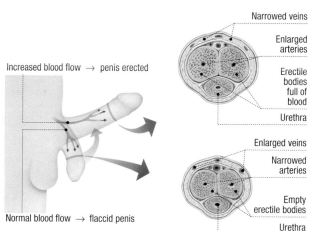

Increased blood flow → penis erected

Normal blood flow → flaccid penis

Narrowed veins

Enlarged arteries

Erectile bodies full of blood

Urethra

Enlarged veins

Narrowed arteries

Empty erectile bodies

Urethra

EJACULATION

Ejaculation consists of the **discharge of semen to the outside**, a reflex act produced involuntarily under control of the sympathetic autonomic nervous system, when a certain **threshold for sexual arousal** is realized. First, there is a rhythmic contraction of the muscles in the walls of the epididymis and in the ductus deferens, which makes the **sperm move forward** to the outside. At the same time, something similar happens in the seminal vesicles and in the prostate, and they empty their contents, so that the sperm and the seminal fluid are directed to the inside of the urethra. In a second phase, some spasmodic contractions of the muscles surrounding the urethra occur. At the same time, the sphincter, which connects this duct with the bladder, contracts, causing the semen to be expelled out, and it gushes out through the urethra to the tip of the penis. This reflex action is usually accompanied by an intense sensation of pleasure, which constitutes the male orgasm.

COMPONENTS OF THE FEMALE REPRODUCTIVE SYSTEM

Uterus

A hollow muscle walled organ covered inside by a mucosa that proliferates in each menstrual cycle. Its role is to receive the fertilized egg and to accommodate the fetus during pregnancy

Ovary

The female gonad; it is in charge of producing ova (gametes or female germinal cells), and it produces female hormones (estrogen and progesterone)

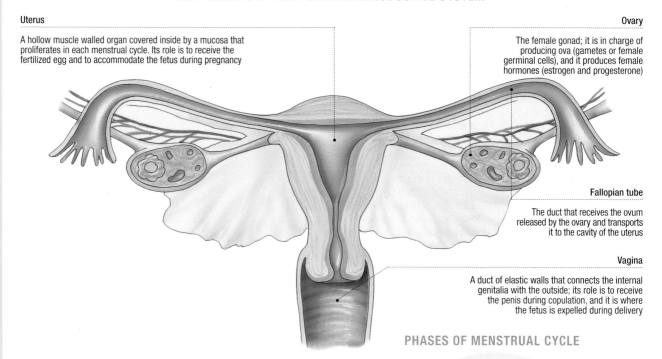

Fallopian tube

The duct that receives the ovum released by the ovary and transports it to the cavity of the uterus

Vagina

A duct of elastic walls that connects the internal genitalia with the outside; its role is to receive the penis during copulation, and it is where the fetus is expelled during delivery

HORMONAL REGULATION OF THE OVARY FUNCTION

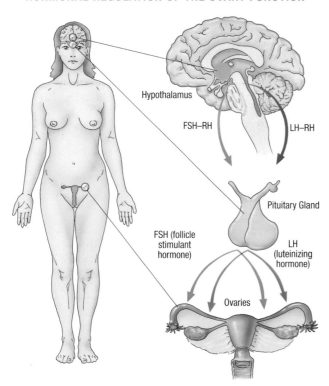

Hypothalamus

FSH–RH

LH–RH

Pituitary Gland

FSH (follicle stimulant hormone)

LH (luteinizing hormone)

Ovaries

Although the menstrual cycle lasts an average of 28 days, the normal duration is between 21 and 35 days.

PHASES OF MENSTRUAL CYCLE

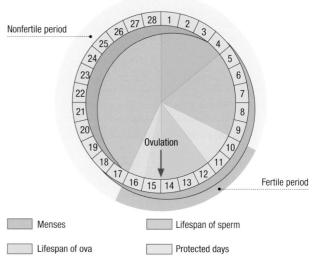

Nonfertile period

Ovulation

Fertile period

Menses

Lifespan of ova

Lifespan of sperm

Protected days

THE MENSTRUAL CYCLE

Under the influence of the hormones of the hypothalamic-pituitary axis, at puberty, the reproductive system starts a **cyclic activity** that continues throughout adult life until menopause. The cycles last approximately **28 days** and are characterized by regular bleeding or **menses**. In each menstrual cycle, the ovaries produce and **release a mature ovum**, ready to be fertilized. At the same time, they **secrete** female **hormones** that **condition the uterus** to receive the fertilized egg if there is one, although they also affect the female's body in different ways. Because the ovum is expelled (**ovulation**) by the middle of the cycle and both the sperm and the ovum have a limited lifespan, it can be said that the menstrual cycle has a **fertile phase**, during which sexual intercourse could lead to a pregnancy and a nonfertile period, during which, in theory, it is more difficult to produce a fertilized egg.

FUNCTIONS OF THE OVARIES

The ovaries have two functions: they are in charge of the **production of ova** and they have an **endocrine activity**. Both functions are regulated by pituitary gonadotrophins. The production of ova starts in puberty, when in a cycle and under the influence of FSH, some of the **primary follicles**, present in the ovaries since birth, start to mature. At the same time, the oocytes or **immature germ cells** contained inside start to mature, too. As the follicles mature, they produce **estrogen**, which prepares the uterus for the possible implantation of a fertilized egg. Generally, only one ovarian follicle matures, while the rest atrophies. Fourteen days into the cycle, the follicle is already mature and bursts onto the surface of the ovary, resulting in ovulation. The oocyte, now turned into an ovum, detaches from the ovary and enters the fallopian tube, where sperm enter in order to fertilize the ovum. Under the influence of LH, the remains of the follicle turn into **corpus luteum** or **yellow** body and continue secreting estrogen. If no eggs are fertilized, the corpus luteum atrophies and turns into **corpus albicans** and stops making hormones, which causes menstruation. And the cycle repeats over and over, as long as no pregnancies take place, until menopause.

At birth, the ovaries have some 400,000 primary oocytes; but, only a few hundred manage to mature during the female's reproductive stage.

UTERINE CHANGES IN THE MENSTRUAL CYCLE

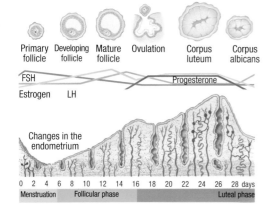

Primary follicle | Developing follicle | Mature follicle | Ovulation | Corpus luteum | Corpus albicans

FSH
Estrogen LH
Progesterone

Changes in the endometrium

0 2 4 6 8 10 12 14 16 18 20 22 24 26 28 days
Menstruation | Follicular phase | Luteal phase

HORMONAL REGULATION OF BREASTFEEDING

Hypothalamus
Pituitary gland
Prolactin
Oxytocin
Nerve impulses
Milk production stimulation
Suckling
Acinus contraction and gland ducts

OVARY ACTIVITY DURING THE MENSTRUAL CYCLE

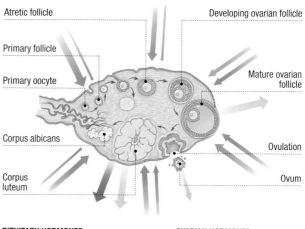

Atretic follicle
Developing ovarian follicle
Primary follicle
Primary oocyte
Mature ovarian follicle
Corpus albicans
Ovulation
Corpus luteum
Ovum

PITUITARY HORMONES
→ FSH
→ LH

OVARIAN HORMONES
→ Estrogens
→ Progesterone

FUNCTION OF THE UTERUS

The uterus has the role of **receiving the fertilized egg** and housing the fetus during pregnancy. It prepares for this with each menstrual cycle, under the influence of female hormones produced by the ovary. In the first part of the cycle, the estrogens secreted by the ovarian follicles give rise to the **proliferative or follicular phase**. In this phase, the mucous layer that covers the inside of the uterus, the **endometrium**, thickens and prepares getting ready for the eventual implantation of a fertilized egg. After ovulation, in the second part of the cycle, the progesterone produced by the corpus luteum gives rise to the **secretory or luteal phase**. In this phase, the endometrium continues to thicken, its glands activate, and its vascularization reaches a maximum. All this is done in preparation for a possible pregnancy. But, if during the cycle there are no fertilized eggs to start a pregnancy and the production of ovarian hormones decreases abruptly, the endometrium **sheds** and the remainder is eliminated, together with blood, through the vagina: this is the **menses**, lasting between three to five days. This usually happens every 28 days.

FUNCTION OF THE BREAST

Breasts are also part of the female reproductive system and have a very special function: to **produce breast milk**, the appropriate food for the newly born. In each menstrual cycle, the breasts prepare for a possible pregnancy, but their development continues only if there is a pregnancy, in which case, **the mammary glands multiply** and acquire appropriate features for producing milk. After delivery, under the influence of the hormone called **prolactin**, the mammary glands activate and start their secretion. When the baby suckles, it causes a stimulus and prolactin is released, and milk production continues during the breastfeeding period. This also causes the release of **oxytocin**, a hormone that causes a contraction of the mammary glands and favors the discharge of milk through the nipple. When breastfeeding ends and the production of prolactin ceases, the mammary glands stop making milk and go back to their prepregnancy resting state.

HUMAN DEVELOPMENT

Growth and development is a complex process, produced by the continuous interaction of **hereditary and environmental factors**. This determines not only an obvious **increase in dimensions** during childhood and puberty but also an **actual transformation** of the body. Adult features appear progressively.

CHANGES PRODUCED IN BODY PROPORTIONS BETWEEN FETAL AND ADULT LIVES

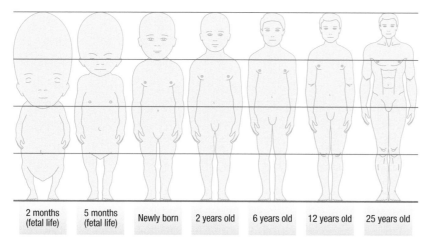

| 2 months (fetal life) | 5 months (fetal life) | Newly born | 2 years old | 6 years old | 12 years old | 25 years old |

Between birth and adulthood, the head grows approximately twice its length, while the trunk grows three times, arms four times, and legs five times. While at 2 months after conception, the head has 50% of the total body length, in adult life it only has 10% of the body size.

MALE DEVELOPMENT DURING PUBERTY

In boys, the first physical change characteristic of puberty is the **enlargement of the testes**. Then, wrinkles appear in the scrotum and a little later pubic hair appears. One or two years later, the **length and thickness of the penis increases**, reaching the dimensions of adult life at the end of two or three years. At the same time, **skeletal development** increases, the body grows, and there is an evident **increase in weight**. There is also a marked increase in the volume of muscles and a broadening of shoulders, which, in contrast with a smaller hip perimeter, conform to the typical **male figure**. During this period, the voice becomes deeper, the pubic hair adopts its rhomboid shape typical of males, and body hair begins to appear, together with a moustache and finally the beard.

MALE DEVELOPMENT DURING PUBERTY

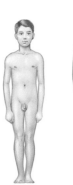
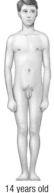
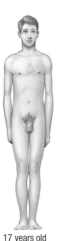

| 11 years old | 14 years old | 17 years old |

FEMALE DEVELOPMENT DURING PUBERTY

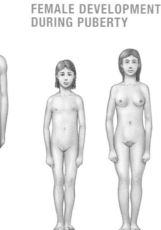
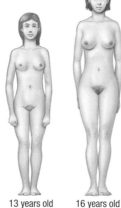

| 9–11 years old | 13 years old | 16 years old |

FEMALE DEVELOPMENT DURING PUBERTY

In girls, the first physical changes in puberty correspond to **breast growth** and the appearance of pubic hair. As breasts continue to grow and pubic hair expands, adopting the triangular shape typical in females, it becomes obvious that the external genitalia grow, and armpit hair appears. The typical teenage growth spurt can be observed and an evident **increase in body weight**, and the female figure is outlined: thighs and hip widen, while fat deposits under the skin increase, bulging especially in buttocks and breasts. A couple of years after the breast changes begin, **menarche** or **first menses** appears. The first menstrual cycles are usually irregular and are not accompanied by ovulation, but as years go by, they become regular and the woman, even though she may look like a teenager, will be ready for the reproductive function.

AGE AT WHICH SOME CHARACTERISTIC CHANGES APPEAR DURING PUBERTY

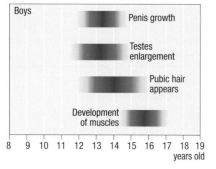

Boys: Penis growth, Testes enlargement, Pubic hair appears, Development of muscles — 8 9 10 11 12 13 14 15 16 17 18 19 years old

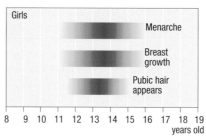

Girls: Menarche, Breast growth, Pubic hair appears — 8 9 10 11 12 13 14 15 16 17 18 19 years old

Introduction

A Perfect Machine

Skin

Digestive System

Nutrition

Respiratory System

Circulatory System and Blood

Nervous System

Musculoskeletal System

Urinary System

Endocrine System

Immune System

The Senses

Genetics

Reproductive System

Human Development

Index

DEVELOPMENT OF BOYS AND GIRLS TO AGE 7

Age	Boys		Girls	
	Size (in)	Weight (lbs)	Size (in)	Weight (lbs)
Birth	19.8	7.7	19.6	7.4
3 mo	23.8	12.5	23.4	12.3
6 mo	26.1	16.7	25.5	16
9 mo	28	20	27.5	19.1
1 yr	29.6	22.2	29.2	21.3
1.5 yrs	32.2	25.1	31.8	24.4
2 yrs	34.4	27.7	34	27.1
2.5 yrs	36.2	29.9	35.9	29.5
3 yrs	37.8	32.1	37.6	31.7
3.5 yrs	39.2	34.3	39.1	33.9
4 yrs	40.7	36.3	40.6	36.1
4.5 yrs	42.5	38.3	42	38.5
5 yrs	43.3	41.4	43	41
5.5 yrs	45	45.6	44.4	44
6 yrs	46.2	48.5	45.6	46.2
6.5 yrs	47.5	51.1	46.8	49.3
7 yrs	48.8	54	48.1	52.2

TEENAGE GROWTH SPURT

If during childhood, the **increase in body size** usually does not exceed 4 cm a year, the beginning of puberty marks a faster rate in the increase in height, with a **speed** that sometimes **doubles** and gives rise to the famous "teenage growth spurt." In girls, the growth spurt usually starts between the ages of 9 and 11, and the peak lasts one or two years, ending toward the age of 15–16, coinciding with the regularization of the menstrual cycle. In boys, however, this usually starts about the age of 12, but it lasts longer and it ends later, between the ages of 17 and 18. This difference in the beginning and the duration of the growth spurt is evident: if girls are taller than boys at the beginning of puberty, after a few years, this tendency reverses.

For the last 150 years, coinciding with the industrial revolution, a significant increase in body size in adults in developed countries has been observed.

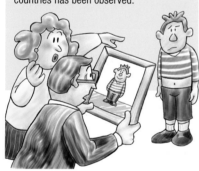

Under normal conditions, puberty starts between the ages of 9 and 13, and it extends, on average, for four years, although physical changes take a few more years to complete.

DEVELOPMENT OF SIZE AND WEIGHT IN PUBERTY

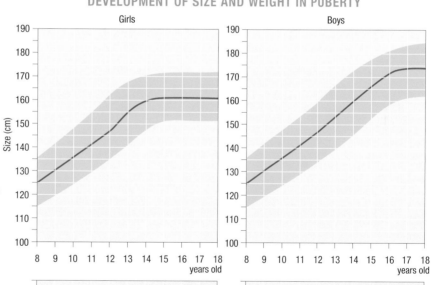

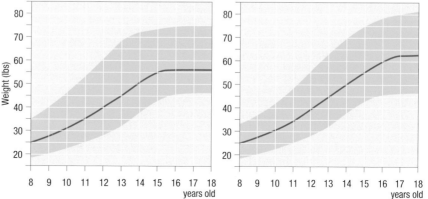

INDEX